What other readers are saying about

THE FIRST MEDICAL PROTOCOL
PRAYER

"Never having had any serious medical issues in our family, past or present, Guy Carbonneau's chronicle, The First Medical Protocol – "Prayer" presents a revealing insight into the physical and emotional drainage that people experience when suddenly faced with a debilitating disease. The toll on the body of the patient, the helpless and empty feelings of family members and friends, the skills and expertise of medical professionals and an abiding faith in a merciful God all interacting with one another provides a "Real Life" traumatic scenario of the events that occur when battling a potentially deadly malady.

This book offers a service to its readers as to the struggles that will be encountered, the hope and optimism that will emerge, and a renewed appreciation for life. It is simultaneously heart wrenching and heart warming, but ultimately recognizes the Power of Prayer in our lives."

William P. Fisher, Ph.D.

• • • • •

"Guy Carbonneau has written a book that chronicles the daily assault that the battle against cancer requires along with the power of prayer as a tangible weapon. This battle is waged with courage, spirit and love. If not for faith and hope, what do we have to sustain us? The power of prayer is the "First Medical Protocol – Prayer."

Heather Menzies Urich

"The book is an amazing witness to the selfless love and complete devotion the author has to his soul mate, Florence his spouse of over fifty-two years. The journey, and how Guy Carbonneau handled its twists and turns, will be lifted up as a beacon of hope for all who face daunting medical challenges. "The First Medical Protocol – Prayer" is a how-to manual for all of us who hold faith in God and pray for His mercy and His healing touch for ourselves, as well as our loved ones. This book is also a model of all that can be accomplished with hope, fortitude and positive thinking."
Kathy Synder, Ph.D.

• • • • •

"I never thought about it very much but it was an awakening to realize there is so much to know about cancer and the treatments for it. About half way through "The First Medical Protocol - Prayer" I recalled how just a few months ago our elected officials in Washington DC were including something called "End of Life Counselors" in bills dealing with health care reform. This offended me, and your book reminded me why. I prefer to stay with the End of Life Counselor I have had since my earliest days. You may have heard of him. He goes by the name of Christ. His friends call him Jesus. You and your wife Florence sought his counsel and He rewarded you. No one can replace Him. Well done."
Stephen J. Kolski

• • • • •

I applaud Guy Carbonneau and his wife for having the courage and selflessness to share their intimate journey with cancer. The insight into the particular diagnosis was educational and heart warming. If I were ever inflicted with this horrible disease, I would want both of them on my side! Guy Carbonneau's phenomenal research and unyielding support of his wife was definitely what carried her through and gave her the strength to carry on even through the days when she was tired, sick or ready to give up. It is inspirational to hear about his unshakeable faith in God. As he says in his story, it is hard to comprehend why God would make one suffer and endure such hardship. The stories he presents about others who had no support system and had endured what seemed like insurmountable odds helped to put my life and difficulties into perspective.
Janine Brisebois

THE FIRST MEDICAL PROTOCOL

PRAYER

When Faith Intersects Science
Miraculous Things Occur

G. P. Carbonneau

Cover and interior design by Jim Becker

Contents

Contents

Contents

To the women who have taught me
How to be a better man - A better husband:
My mother, Yvette,
My daughters-in-law, Janet and Vickie
And, especially my wife, Florence.

Acknowledgments

To my spiritual advisors, Rev. John Bluett, and Rev. George Dunne, of St. Stephen Catholic Community, - your enjoyable and inspiring homilies have opened my eyes and heart to the Bible Scriptures. In the course of your gracious words of welcome, to the Catholic Community of St. Stephen, all have been touched by your grace and all continue to grow spiritually. The St. Stephen Catholic Community is blessed to have you both. Thank you, and God Bless you.

To my St. Stephen Chapel friends and Bread Angels. Your "Amazing Grace" has and continues to inspire me to be a better person - Thank you...

In Florence's Own Words

Although this story is about my wife's journey, it is written from a husband's perspective – mine. Much of the story evolved from my emails, the responses to those emails and my research on the fundamental principles of breast cancer. However, the most important ingredient to this story was to reveal Florence's feelings as she traveled her incredible journey. To do this, and to understand her feelings, you will find "In Florence's Words" throughout the book. The source of the many thoughts, the feelings, the good times, and the bad times are from her own diary, a diary she kept throughout her journey – and in her own words.

To My Dear Wife, Florence

I still need to find more ways to express my love and appreciation to you. Your courage and spirit continue to amaze me. The loving notes from everyone tell me how much you continue to be an inspiration to so many. Nothing, not even cancer, will ever defeat the love we share. It will never tear the bonds we both have forged together over all these years by this fearful experience.

Introduction

We live in a weary world, endlessly peppered with news of suffering, transgressions, man's inhumanity to man and to the world he calls home. At times, the darkness can overwhelm us, pull us into its grip and leave us wondering if the light is still there, if it is still available to us. And then, a new melody comes across the radio, a fire-red sunrise blazes across the horizon, we turn to find the unexpected smile of a stranger, or we read a story that redefines love, and for a time our hearts are lifted, the light is rediscovered and the darkness lifts.

This is a book that intensifies that light; that cannot help but brighten your day. Yes, it is a story of a woman with cancer and her valiant struggle against this insidious disease. And it is the story of her husband's struggle to remain strong when, for the first time in his life, he is powerless to help.

But it is also more than that. It is the story of two people committed to remaining a light to each other (and to the world around them) regardless of their suffering. It is about their refusal to be pulled into the darkness and the myriad ways in which the world responds to that commitment by delivering more love and light to their journey. Strangers emerge; family responds, the disease retreats and, most important, God emerges as never before. We are told in ways large and small that the light, in fact, never left us, but that, at times, we must experience the darkness to remember.

On a practical level, it is Guy Carbonneau, the entrepreneur, the engineer, the man, dealing with the disease the only way he knows how: by conducting extensive research into his wife's malady and her medical regimen, and then using that knowledge to keep us informed. It is Florence's grace, humor, and dignity in her own words, in battling the disease, the pain, the exhaustion, and the fear - always the fear. And it is this extraordinary couple's commitment to facing the disease together, of finding laughter wherever and whenever it can be had. It is Florence taking strength in her faith and of Guy redefining his own.

Ultimately, the book reminds us that it is in suffering that we are reminded of our gifts, and that where light exists darkness cannot abide.

Amazing Grace - "How Sweet The Sound

The words above may make some of you think I'm embarking in an area that may be uncomfortable for you. What does "Amazing Grace - how sweet the sound" have to do with Florence and my coping with her diagnosis of breast cancer, and the resultant chemo and radiation therapy? I want to be very clear and say to the readers, that the use of my spiritual beliefs and practices to cope with this very stressful time in my life has been an unbelievably rewarding experience.

Everybody needs somebody or something to sustain him or her through the bad times. For me, it is my Christian faith. My religious expression has, and continues to be, the mental mechanism that helps me put a more positive spin on Florence's diagnosis of breast cancer and her ultimate fate. I think that the prayer talk has provided me with relief of stress that is not attainable by other forms of talk. Florence's diagnosis has propelled me on a spiritual trek, which by many accounts, it usually does. From time to time this book will be riddled with faith-based dialogue, and from time to time you will often read that prayers to the Great Physician were a vital component to Florence's cancer treatment protocol.

So, to the doubting Thomas (reader) you are free to put this book down and go about your business. If, however, "Amazing Grace" and Breast Cancer intrigue you, then continue reading.

Before you do, I must first thank the excellent team of doctors who cared for my wife, Florence, and who always took the time for one more question.

Jon D. Wiese, MD, FACS - General Surgery
Sonalee K. Shroff, MD - Oncologist
David A. Diamond, MD - Radiation Oncology
Dr. Christian Kovats, D.O., P.A.
Meredith Luce, MS, RD, LD/N – Nutritionist

I am grateful to all the breast cancer experts who spent time with me in person and on the phone. I would especially like to thank my dear and long time friend and confidante, Dr. Robert Baratta, who always had the time to field a medical query. Also, a very big loving hug to Dr. Jan Jablonski who helped Florence and me form the medical team. Her expertise was invaluable.

I cannot thank God enough for the wonderful and inspiring support given to Florence and me by our sons, Guy Anthony and Clinton James, their wives, Janet and Vickie, and our grandchildren, Joshua, Jordan, Jessica, and Amanda. Their love for Florence and me was the greatest gift of all throughout Florence's journey. They continue to be a pillar of strength to us.

AND, then there are those special family members and friends I want to thank. This very supportive group kept me on the right track with their honest and intuitive feelings.

July 3rd - The Journey Begins

"Guy, I have a lump." With those five words, our lives were forever changed.

Following an extended visit with some family in Phoenix, Florence and I had just arrived home in Orlando where we were scheduled to undergo routine physical examinations. Although it was necessary for us to have the physicals after more than six months on the road, we were more excited to see our children and grandchildren.

Earlier that spring Florence had detected a lump in her left breast, a development that did not wholly alarm us but created an understandable uneasiness in Florence. Over the succeeding days Florence found herself continually feeling for the lump, a distraction that potentially posed a serious health risk but counterbalanced by her overall good health. "Nothing to worry about," she told herself, and I was only too happy to concur.

She would ask me to feel for it, and often I struggled to locate it. Even when I did, at times I was uncertain if "it" was actually there. By the next week the lump appeared to have disappeared, allowing us both to breathe a bit easier and sink back into the joys of our travels.

The next few days she continued to self-diagnose her breast for any changes. She even had me feel for the lump again, but I had difficulty in finding the exact location and could not tell if indeed, there was anything out of the ordinary.

The next week she could not find the lump and wondered if what she had felt was anything to be concerned about. Knowing she had not had a mammogram for some years, she realized it was time to get a thorough physical. She also made appointments for me, as I too had not had a physical in a long time.

In Florence's Own Words

"We were in Scottsdale, Arizona visiting my brother and his wife when I said to Guy "it's time to take a break and go home to see the kids and grandkids, and get some medical stuff done".

Not for any special reason, but it had been a few years since we had any physicals, and me a mammogram. We've been staying with Ken and Susan for several months. Ken was preparing for Deep Brain Stimulation (DBS) surgery to help control some of his Parkinson's problems. So we made our plans to take a break, and left on July 2nd to head home. Our plan was to be back in time for Ken's surgery."

The following day, July 3rd, Florence's first regular check-up was for a mammogram - her first in three years. The news wasn't good. The results indicated some concern by the doctors and the need for further tests. A sonogram was ordered immediately, and two days later the sonogram was taken. I sat in the waiting room thinking, "What is happening? Is this for real? My best friend, - life partner, is in another room, without me, finding out if the lump in her body is really bad. I have to be strong. I have to be there for the person I care more about than anything in the world.

Finally, a nurse came out and asked me to come back to the diagnostic room. I entered a semi-dark room with black and white monitors everywhere. Florence and the doctor stood in front of a monitor with symbols, white outlines and markings, all indicating something was not right. As I approached Florence, I've never seen her as scared as she was that morning.

The radiologist looked at both of us, and then looked back at the images on the screen, and with five little words introduced us to the world of breast cancer: "Looks like cancer to me."

With tears in both of our eyes, we said nothing; we just held each other knowing this was not good. I felt ashamed not to have any words for her. I was - so - emotional. I needed to know how to comfort her when her face looked more sorrowful than I'd had ever recalled it being. "Sorrow" was not a typical emotion for her.

Our lives were being turned upside down. Deep inside I was shocked and scared. I stared at the monitor, then at the ceiling, trying to absorb everything while trying to avoid the stark medical reality. Does Florence have breast cancer? If the radiologist was correct,

I could not imagine how Florence and I would cope in the months ahead.

The doctor told us a biopsy would be necessary to see if "the lump" was malignant. How could it be malignant when there was no history of cancer in her family? I was the only one with a family history of cancer. I guess we cling to whatever hopes we feel available.

In Florence's Own Words

"On July 3rd my first appointment was for my mammogram. When I was done and ready to leave, the technician came out and said that my Primary Care doctor wanted to see me right away. I went over to his office with Guy and he told me I needed to have a sonogram right away as I had a very sizeable lump that did not look good. My heart just sank, but started thinking it's probably just a cyst and I'm not going to worry about it, at least I thought I wasn't going to worry about it.

Two very long days later, I had the sonogram and the nurse said the radiologist wanted to talk to me. I went in to see him and he told me it looked like breast cancer. When he showed me the sonogram I could see a spread of what looked like sparkled dots. It hit me what he had just said, "Breast Cancer." Of course, I lost it. You never expect anyone to be saying that to you, maybe to someone else, but not me. Guy was in the waiting room and I felt so bad to have to tell him about this since his mom and two sisters had breast cancer and two of them passed away. His other sister is a breast cancer survivor. They went and got him, I could hardly look at him, but he came over and hugged me right away. He knew! That was a hug I can still feel to this day. What an incredible shock, for the both of us. I'll never forget that day, or those words, "breast cancer." Thank God I have Guy, I could not have handled it myself.

The hardest thing I had to do was tell the kids, and it was really hard. They were absolutely wonderful, as usual. Their support started that very moment and has not stopped. (I love them all so much) I asked them to tell the grandkids. I just couldn't do that. I knew I would fall apart if I had to tell them. I just didn't want them to worry.

Right away Clint started researching Breast Cancer. He was involved with the Leukemia Society, and started calling the doctors he knew. He was incredibly helpful. We got second opinions and suggestions right away. Guy also called Dr. Jan Jablonski, a long time friend of our family."

Fifty-Five Years Ago - Boy Meets Girl

Recently, I had the urge to look through the high school yearbook, causing me to reminisce about memories of long ago. The school at that time was six years old, and the attendance was about three hundred and fifty students - all boys. Yes, Curley was an all boys' school, but less than a mile away was an all girls' school, Notre Dame Academy.

I attended Archbishop Curley High School in Miami, Florida, during the fifties. I was a combination of a rebel and a jock. In school I remember rebelling against everything I felt I was forced to learn, those things I didn't believe would apply to my life. I was definitely an underperformer, and never took a book home with me during my senior year. Somehow, I managed to graduate.

During my three years at Curley, I would often think of ways to beat the system. At that time, I had a strong interest in electronics, and would often repair the neighbors' radios. I remember being challenged to create a one-way communication system from me to a student friend attending a class Vocabulary Bee. I cut out the inside pages of a book and placed a telephone mouthpiece and electronics inside. The classroom teacher would not know what was going on. Before the class started I installed a wire from my desk, in the back of the room, to my classmate sitting at his desk, in the front of the room. I gave him a telephone earpiece wrapped in a handkerchief. The handkerchief was to disguise the earpiece when placed next to his ear. When the teacher gave him a word I would look up the definition, and in a very low voice I would give him the answer via the earpiece in his handkerchief. He would then repeat the answer to the teacher. The teacher was having difficulty believing that this student, my friend, was able to answer the questions he asked of him. Apparently, he thought, out of the group who participated, he should have failed much earlier. My friend would have been number one in the contest, but it seemed the acoustics of the room were changing. Not sure why. As a result, a whistle sound was generated in my friend's earpiece causing him to frown, with a facial expression of pain. Not good! Occasionally, the teacher hearing the noise would look around the room to see where it was coming from. Scared I would be found out, I quickly turned off the electronics. Even though there were problems, my friend finished second in the Vocabulary Bee. The teacher never did find out what was going on. However, my physics teacher did, and he was so impressed with how I put everything together, he gave me an "A" in his class. Better than that, I was able to restore my mom's home telephone. Not bad, huh?

Curley High School had always boasted a top-notch football team in the Miami area. Our small school would compete with schools whose population exceeded two thousand students. In spite of the size, our football team would outperform them on the gridiron. One of the main reasons our athletes were spectacular performers was because they were playing for a phenomenal coach - Armand "Stitch" Vari. Stitch, as he was often called, gave me a chance to try out for a spot on the football team. He was a demanding coach and interested in his players. He was interested in me, and I would become one of his starters. During my junior year, six seniors went on to earn college football scholarships. The colleges knew they were getting athletes who were well coached and had high self-discipline, a trademark of Coach Vari. Playing football for Coach Vari was a most rewarding and wonderful experience for me, and my teammates. It would be years later that I would renew a closer relationship with Coach Vari and his wife, Jacque. We continue to this day to be good friends.

It was during the fall of 1959 when I met my wife Florence. A high school buddy, Steve Kolski, introduced me to her. He told me that Florence was moving into the area and that she was somewhat distraught at having to leave Nutley High School, in New Jersey. He told me she would be attending Notre Dame Academy for Girls. He invited me to double date with him and one of Florence's cousins, Lois Hyland. I accepted, and that became the most momentous decision I would ever make in my life. The events of that evening were, well, incredible.

I didn't entirely feel normal or comfortable at first, especially when I tried to engage her in conversation, but I could see that something was working, so I kept at it. Every now and then I would catch her staring at me. I didn't react, but just kept saying to myself, "Boy, am I glad I'm here."

Thank you, Lois and Steve, for introducing me to the love of my life. Because of you we found each other. With God's help, our future will always be with each other. [54]I cannot express my thanks enough to the both of you.

A Day at Curley High School

Florence had a brother who chose not to continue his seminary studies for the priesthood for personal reasons and applied for a teaching position at Curley. Mr. Hyland, as the students would respectfully call him, could easily be mistaken for a student rather than a teacher as he walked the hallways of Curley. Being concerned he may be picked on by other students; my friend and I were obliged to escort him to his class each morning. We also gave him the first parking spot in the parking lot. We didn't tell him it belonged to the Dean of Boys.

I remember Mr. (Jim) Hyland's first day when he entered the classroom, and before he started an opening prayer, he turned and faced the crucifix above the blackboard. At the end of the class session, and before dismissal, he again turned, faced the crucifix, and said a closing prayer. When he turned back to dismiss the students, the classroom was empty. All the students left the classroom via the backdoor leaving him alone - in prayer. His first week at Curley was stressful; I'm sure. One more thing, Mr. Hyland often would double date with Florence and me. In those instances, I would call him Jim, his first name. Can you believe that? How many high school teachers do you know would go out on dates with a student and his girlfriend? I'm not sure, but I think he gave me a "C" minus in his class. Oops!

Over the next few months, Florence and I would spend hours together, going to the movies, picnics at the local beaches with her family, high school-dances, everything normal high school teens do, at least in those days.

Florence grew up in a family filled with love. She had three brothers and two sisters. As I look back, what kept her family together was the respect and trust they had for each other. Relationships within families are not always easy, particularly as people grow older. However, Florence's family had and continues to have a wonderful relationship. I've had the wonderful opportunity over the years to be a part of this family. Her mom and dad were great, especially her dad. My buddy warned me earlier, that Florence's dad was a big fan of football. He had played semi-pro football in New Jersey, and he loved watching Notre Dame on TV. All of this was good for me as I played high school football and that became a general topic of discussion with us. One of my most vivid memories was when, in her exuberance, Florence fell through the bleachers watching me score a touchdown. From there, the romance really began to blossom. It felt right from the start. I still smile when I think of that first kiss. Time was slipping away so fast; I really wanted the clock to stop so I could really enjoy those moments with her.

Some would say our first great love occurred sometime in our teens, but I would say it occurred when we first married, still young, fresh, optimistic and ready for life. It's the first time you learn to communicate with another person, and if you want the relationship to last it's when both partners share fundamental beliefs. They say good relationships are built on time-tested foundations, one of which is you have to spend time with each other.

Our Commitment

We were married in Miami, Florida, at St. Mary's Cathedral on July 15, 1961. Florence and I both made a commitment that wonderful day, a defining trait of our marriage. It was a commitment to stay together the rest of our lives. We took the words, "for better or for worse," very seriously. The ceremony was exciting for us and our family and friends. We were Mr. Right and Mrs. Right, dancing to our song, "Lavender Blue."

The marriage brought us two boys. First, Guy Anthony arrived, and then Clinton James, both absolutely wonderful gifts from God who would bring us joy and amazement. Giving birth is the most painful and yet incredible event a woman will ever experience (my opinion, of course). I was so proud and respectful of Florence, and overcome by the process of bringing new life into this world.

I was so excited. I was going to teach them everything: integrity, honor, how to win, and how to lose. They were going to do everything with us, as a family. I was going to exist for three human beings - fantastic! Unbelievable! It's the best thing that has ever happened to me. They had become my life I had become their life.

During the first years of our marriage, we opened ourselves up to everything that love can bring to our marriage: communication, sincerity, and passion. Was it easy? Not always! We both learned together in love, and a continuing commitment to keep together - always.

Our story seems unique to us and yet is the same as every love story out there. I wish everyone could experience the happiness and fun we've been having. When you're doing everything right as a couple, you know you're doing things right!

The next fifty-two years were filled with incredible experiences. Watching the boys grow from adolescents into young adults and eventually into married life, were the most rewarding parts of our journey. The boys, our young men, married two wonderful ladies, Vickie and Janet. Florence and I fell in love with them immediately. We were fortunate that the boys married two people who brought with them the same core beliefs that our family shared, a tribute to their parents, no doubt.

"If I had known grandkids were going to be so much fun, I would have had them first." Where have I heard that before? Yes, indeed, it happened - as expected. Grandkids! They joined us starting with Joshua, Jordan, Jessica and finally, Amanda Grace. I believe God made the family structure so we could be grandma and grandpa to our grandchildren. We get to start all over again, raising children. Okay, maybe I've gone too far.

Well, they say a family who prays together stays together. For as long as I can remember this family has prayed together and, to this day, stayed together. It is a joy and sometimes emotional for me to sit with the grandkids, daughters-in-law, my two sons and my wife altogether in the same pew at a Sunday mass. This is truly a family I am so proud of and grateful to have in my life.

Cancer History and Me

I have been blessed to have two sisters. One who died of breast cancer at the age of fifty-four; the other who is alive and well, and is now an 18 year breast cancer survivor. Thankfully, people do survive!

My Mother was the first to be diagnosed with breast cancer. I was a young teen at the time and had no idea what this dreaded disease was all about. At the moment I'm not sure I really knew she had cancer. All I knew was that she was sick, and our house was filled with turmoil for about a year.

My mother had a radical mastectomy involving the removal of both of the two chest muscles, as well as the breast and lymph nodes. The strain of major surgery on my mother had to affect her physical and emotional wellbeing. With the loss of mom's breasts, it had to bring feelings of depression and insecurities. Also, in my mom's case, there was no breast-conserving therapy performed. Mom had two more recurrences of cancer. The final one took her life at the age of ninety. So, who has the history? I have the history, not my wife Florence.

Familial cancer has always been in the back of my mind. I also knew that these vicious cancers might have hereditary causes, but there was never any hard evidence, and so I personally never took the time to get medical advice or get a physical. I did read that a blood test could be performed to see who carries the BRCA1 or BRCA2 gene mutation in a family who has a history of cancer. Through diagrams and studies, doctors can trace the gene back to family members.

It was explained to me how gene mutation can disable the tumor-fighting ability in particular parts of the body. This gives women an eighty-five percent chance of developing breast cancer, as well as other cancers. Being positive for this gene also means there is a fifty-percent chance that you will pass the gene on to your children. Had my mother performed this analysis it would have been clear that there was a fifty-percent chance of my sisters also having this genetic defect; thereby, solving the mystery of why cancer had invaded my family for so many years. The reality is the test wasn't available to my mom, and cancer did indeed strike to take my sister at an early age and, later, my Mom. It also invaded my older sister who survived because of a great team of doctors, a very positive mental attitude, and prayers from everyone.

This horrific disease had invaded my sisters, my mom, and now my wife. I am constantly aware of the possibility that I am next. A very scary proposition for sure.

Time for a Biopsy

Florence's lump was detected through a mammogram and a self-exam, and now it was time for a biopsy to learn if the lesion is benign or malignant. On July sixth, I drove Florence to the Florida Hospital Mammography Center. My thoughts were, "Maybe it's a false alarm; perhaps the tumor is benign." Just because the doctor wants Florence to have a biopsy does not mean she has breast cancer. Most breast lumps are not cancerous. However, I knew having a biopsy, the removal and testing of a suspicious area of the breast would be the only way to know for sure.

The doctor started the surgical biopsy by first administering anesthesia delivered by an IV. Florence gradually entered a twilight sleep. The surgeon removed a part of the lesion and readied the specimen for a pathologist who would assess it for cancerous cells. During the procedure, and knowing what was happening, I couldn't sit still in the waiting room. I needed to do something. The fear of breast cancer brought with it concerns and discomforting emotions, anxieties, uncertainty. I felt I was out of control. I had a strong urge to leave the Mammography Center and find a church to pray.

I knew that nearby there was a Catholic church, St. Margaret Mary, where one of our sons had been married. I drove to the church hoping it would be open. Fortunately, the nearest door to where I was parked was open. I went inside and knelt down in a pew. The church was empty and extremely quiet. The silence was eerie, yet peaceful. Colorful shadows emanated from the pillars and walls. The light from the stained glass windows reflected off the newly polished tile floors in all of the colors of the rainbow. It was quite serene. A perfect place to pray! Who said that I couldn't bow to prayer? I believed in the work the medical doctors were doing, and I would follow all the instructions they gave. But, I also knew that the Great Physician was above and I could talk to Him. How do I talk to Him? What do I say? There have been so many times that I felt I couldn't pray. It has always been difficult for me to get the right words out of my mouth - and from my heart.

I understand from my upbringing that prayer is incredibly important to enjoy an intimate relationship with God. I was taught that through prayer you could obtain God's assurance for every situation.

Now was the time for me to have a life changing conversation with God, but how? In this time of need how do I cry out for God's help? I'm overwhelmed with my first emotional eruption, or what some people call a meltdown. I'm alone with no one to comfort me. All I can think of is Florence. I struggle to keep the tears back while staring at the altar, and the crucifix above. I think of the rosary.

In my Catholic upbringing, I was taught to pray the rosary. It was something we did in Catholic school as well as at home. In my younger days I found myself often reciting the rosary mostly in times of difficulty. It seems we "resort" to prayer when temporal things fail.

The rosary is marvelous in its simplicity. The word rosary comes from Latin and means a garland of roses, the rose being one of the flowers used to symbolize the Virgin Mary. Even Protestants now say the rosary, recognizing it as a truly biblical form of prayer. The prayers that comprise it actually come from the Bible! I remember that through the rosary, the faithful will receive abundant grace, as though from the very hands of the Mother of the Redeemer. However, it's been a very long time since I've said one. I'm not sure I remember how to start and would I be able to complete the whole rosary without being overwhelmed with emotions? Slowly, I managed to start with the sign of the cross and continued until the last prayer was said. I ended by knowing that the Lord will work out His perfect will in Florence's situation and bring about healing. I asked The Great Physician to heal her from the biopsy procedure and, if there is cancer, to remove it from her body.

I left the church feeling the holy place I had entered allowed me to pour out the contents of my heart with honesty. I was able to send the world away in order to create a space where I could pray to the God who was waiting for me. I was in the sheer silence of my own solitude and able to use my own private words. I had no desire to leave the house of prayer, but I had to be with Florence. God was near!

As I entered the Mammography Center Florence was being escorted to the waiting room; two nurses were holding her gently. For a brief moment we stared at each other. Staring into her eyes my reaction were feelings of sadness, shock and fear. What was to happen next to her? I tried not to speculate, but my emotions did.

This was a time for me to react calmly, to be reassuring, and to keep my emotions in check. But my reflexes took over. Was she in pain? "How are you, Hon?" I said. I hated to see my Florence in pain. "Is everything okay?" She was pale and still a little groggy. She answered, "I'm okay. Everything went well."

The doctor said that the results would be available to Florence's oncologist and surgeon by the following Tuesday. After some of the grogginess wore off, Florence was released and I took her home.

The biopsy results were due on Tuesday, July Tenth. The next few days were filled with questions and fraught with anxiety. A significant part of the fear of breast cancer diagnosis is the uncertainty and the feeling that we're losing control of our lives. We're being swept away on a journey that we don't want to take. It's hard to imagine how anything good could happen over all of this. This certainly will be a test of Florence's optimism and confidence.

In Florence's Own Words

"The biopsy results showed I definitely had Breast Cancer, and not a very good kind. I was still in complete shock. Had to have several tests done. Not sure of exact date. I met with an Oncologist, and Guy and I both liked her a lot. Her name is Dr. Sonalee Shroff. She seems to be very smart and we've heard through the grapevine she is one of the best. So, so far so good! Lucky me."

Time to Tell The Family

Telling the family and friends about Florence's diagnosis would be a challenging experience for the both of us. It would be stressful and more emotional than the actual diagnosis. However, going through the breast cancer diagnosis with only Florence and my knowing would be worse. We had to think about the family and their feelings, in addition to those of our friends. It was necessary to tell them, even though it would be difficult. I didn't want them to find out from someone else long after we knew.

Whom should we tell first? It was obvious. We would tell our children first. After getting the news from the doctor we drove to our son Clint's house. I was walking to the front door when Vickie, Clint's wife, came out to greet me. I looked at her and she looked at me - no words were said. She knew this was not good news when she saw the tears in my eyes. Vickie quickly wrapped her arms around Florence. They didn't have to say anything. I went inside the house and met Clint, stared at him, trying to give him the news. It was difficult. He also knew it was not good news. Even though this was a terrifying experience, I tried hard not to pass on the sense of overwhelming anxieties I was feeling. We talked to the both of them, at the same time, trying to remember all the details given to us by the doctors. Later that evening we met with Guy Anthony and his wife Janet, along with Clint and Vickie, at a local restaurant, and there we gave them the news. The four of them sensed how scared we both were even though we tried to convey calmness and optimism. The biggest challenge was saying the words, "Mom has cancer." Saying those words to the kids released emotions that I had been trying to suppress. It was at that time I said to myself I would never break down in front of them. I would hold my composure when I was with them. And so, as a result, I spent a lot of time in a bathroom with the door locked.

I know the diagnosis itself scares them, but I also know they understand what cancer is. All of them including the grandchildren were always by my mom when she struggled with cancer, and they were by my side when my mom finally succumbed to this disease.

Both of our sons are so much alike. They both share common likes and dislikes. Their temperaments are very similar. They are happy, and cheerful, and full of life. They rarely cry. However, they are different in their own ways, too.

Guy Anthony, for the most part, is cautious. He does not like change. He likes order and structure. When he was told the news it was not unusual for him to be extremely quiet, keeping his emotions inside himself. To look at his face that evening, was heartbreaking. His expression of concern and his expression of disbelief were heart wrenching for me. I wanted to tell him, "Guy; I'll fix this, no problem, it will be okay, - I promise."

Clint was different, his reaction was one of deep concern, and sadness by what he knew his mom would be soon going through. He was a lot like me; he needed to fix the problem, move ahead with whatever it would take to remove this foreign invader from our family. His head was already spinning, thinking and looking for something he could do. Already he started to do his own research about cancer on the Internet. He was aggressive, determined he would formulate a plan of attack. He said, "Dad, I want to call my friends at the Leukemia Society for recommendations on whom would be the best doctor to treat mom." Of course I concurred.

"Yes, Clint, that would be excellent."

Guy and Clint are two very special guys who were conceived by two people who loved each other very much. The connection our sons have with us is a bond that can never be broken. We have always loved them both for who they were, and for who we all are when we're together.

They love their wives and children very much and they spend precious time with them. As brothers, they participate in family activities. In this way they keep our family as a priority in their lives. They knew Florence's treatments would bring some unpleasant surprises and probably would result in changes to our family routines. Our schedules will have to be rearranged and any planned travels will be postponed or cancelled for at least a while.

Now it was time to tell Florence's brothers, sisters, my sister, and our friends. Would our family and friends experience anger and depression, or would they overcompensate with positive and upbeat feelings? Florence was great in this area. She immediately chose to call her brothers and sisters. I would be able to talk to them later.

When I did talk to them about the diagnosis, I had to keep control of my emotions; at least I thought I did. What I was afraid of was that some people might not be able to handle the information. It would be better to tell them without going through any emotional breakdown, or pessimism.

I understood that people might not know what to say and could say things that seem insensitive. I learned quickly there really isn't a correct way to deal with the news of telling someone my wife has breast cancer. So, when I did tell our family and friends, I accepted all of their different reactions. Still it was very difficult to deal with something like cancer. I needed to cry but tried hard not to. I was macho, tough - yeah right! Yet, somehow it seemed natural to cry. Some very special people were very supportive, as though they were facing the same situation as I was. It may have been because the person cared about us that they also became upset. Either way I felt it brought us closer together and I was glad I had shared this with them.

I also learned that emails were the best way to communicate with everyone. So I decided to send my first email with the announcement that Florence was diagnosed with breast cancer.

The following was what I said,

"By now all of you have heard from Florence regarding the news from her Doctor. Florence and I came to Florida to take advantage of some normal precautionary medical physicals, and as a result Florence's breast exam turned out positive. Florence and I are moving very quickly on a plan that will give Florence the best treatment available for her. At this time we are establishing a knowledgebase on this insidious disease, and we will pick a treatment protocol based on all of the input given to us. The protocol will be a plan we both feel will treat Florence's cancer. We're both aware that the same type of cancer and the same treatment, may not work the same way for others.

There are very good people out there who are now aware of Florence's condition and will be advising us. The first event is, Florence will need surgery as soon as possible to remove the tumor and to ascertain if her cancer has spread. I'll keep you posted on when.

On another front, this whole ordeal has had a devastating effect on our immediate family, however, Guy A., Clint, Janet and Vickie are committed to the team and all will play an important role, including the grandkids.

Sometimes it's not easy for me to talk about what I feel about all of this. It is indeed difficult, to say the least. Please don't be offended if we fail sometimes to call or not share all of the information with you. We promise we will try our very best to keep you informed.

As many of you know, making a commitment in our family is a very big thing. No matter what the commitment is about! To give up requires no commitment. Fighting this battle will mean a complete change of our lifestyle and leaving our comfort zone. There will be doctors doing things Florence might not like. There will be lots of work for Florence to do. There might even be some pain and suffering. She'll decide that the end is worth it. She is the only one who can do it. No one else will do it for her. There will be no half way. It will be all the way. We have made the commitment. There will be pleasant experiences. There will be unpleasant experiences.

Now this is what we need from you, and it is the easiest contribution you can make. Prayers! "The First Protocol." Your commitment to this is part of Florence's treatment protocol. We accept all types of prayers: long ones and short ones, whatever. You decide."

There were moments during this eventful week when I would look around and just absorb the power emanating from my family. It overwhelmed me when I saw how we all came together as a family. We were one in our hearts, and in a common bond for Florence, my wife, and my kids' mom.

In Florence's Own Words

"I called my brothers and sisters, five of them, (except Ken - I knew I would cry when I talked to him because of what he was already going through, so I asked Guy to make that phone call) and told them I had breast cancer. I didn't cry, and in fact I felt pretty strong, because I didn't want them to worry. They all sounded pretty somber and didn't say a whole lot. I know they were probably as shocked as I was.

We went back to Scottsdale, AZ to get our RV to drive back to Florida. I asked the doctors for the time to drive the RV back and I'm so glad we did that. It gave both of us the time for all of this to sink in. I really felt bad for Guy he looked so worried.

My brother's surgery went very well and we were so glad we were there with him and Susan. A few days before leaving their place, I looked at Ken standing in the kitchen and he was looking quite down; I knew it had to do with his Parkinson's. I said, "Ken can you believe the two of us right now, you with Parkinson's and me with breast cancer? Did you ever believe these days would come?" He just looked at me and came right over and gave me the biggest hug. We stayed there for what felt like about a minute. I knew there were tears in my eyes and I'm sure in his. It was a very memorable moment for me. The ride back to Florida was great, but all the way I just dreaded getting there, knowing what was in store for Guy and me.

It started right away, lots of tests, PET scans, Bone scans, MUGGA scans, CT scans, MRIs, blood tests, etc., etc."

My First Visit To St. Stephen Chapel

On the early morning of Friday, July 6th, after an evening filled with anxieties, and not able to sleep I finally got out of bed, dressed and left the house. Normally my daily ritual was to have coffee at one of the local coffee houses, read a newspaper and "think." Today was different! I decided to visit our local parish church, St, Stephen's, which conducted a Mass each morning at seven AM. It was 6:45, so I drove over to the church and attended the service. It had been a very long time since I attended mass so early in the morning. The sun was just starting to rise, and there were squirrels playing in the large oak trees nearby as I walked toward the chapel door. The morning was quiet, and there were a few people walking toward the entrance of the chapel. I was going into a church again. My first thought was, "why?" Later I would learn it was an opportunity for me to get away from everyone. It was my quiet space, a place to be emotional, to pray, or think about nothing - about everything. It was a wonderful opportunity to pray for Florence. I left the chapel energized and ready for whatever the day would bring. Since that first day, and every morning thereafter, I've attended the 7:00 Mass at St. Stephen's chapel.

After the service, there was an opportunity to meet Fr. George Dunne, the parish priest, and bring him up to date on all of the recent events. He placed one hand on my shoulder and said a few comforting words ending with a suggestion for a healing service on behalf of Florence. He agreed to hold the service at my son's home the following day.

I had told the family the journey Florence is on would have many unpleasant experiences. But there will also be uplifting experiences. The very next day, Saturday, July 7th the house was filled with an unbelievable presence of comfort and love. Everyone felt it. The beautiful table settings my daughters-in-law prepared, the conversations, the humor, the laughter from the grandchildren, and then the Healing Service.

The Healing Service was a spirit-filled blessing for all of us. It offered an opportunity to engage in the ceremony together as a family, sharing a sense of peace even in the midst of Florence's difficulty. It was a spiritual healing as well as a physical healing. There was a feeling of being cared for by God. It made all of us realize the importance of friends and loved ones as a source of comfort and support. This indeed was a pleasant experience for Florence and me, and all of our family.

In Florence's Own Words

"Fr. George came over to Guy and Janet's, and all the kids and grandkids were there. Just looking at Guy, the kids and grandkids, and even Jake the dog during this, just overwhelmed me. I cried at how blessed and lucky I was and felt this strength come over me, that I was going to make it through this. I felt something really overpowering that day. Fr. George was wonderful and I felt so comforted by him."

The next day, after Sunday morning Mass, we stopped to visit with my son, his wife and our grandchildren. As we entered the house, Florence's brothers, sisters, and spouses greeted us. This was a big surprise for Florence and me, and of course the tears were flowing as Florence hugged them all.

The kids had invited Florence's brothers and sisters and their spouses unbeknownst to us. They had prepared appetizers in the afternoon and then a beautiful dinner. Guy Anthony, Janet, Clint & Vickie cooked, cleaned, and waited on us. It was a wonderful experience for Florence to have her sisters, brothers, and spouses with her. It also made it so much easier on Florence, because she hadn't seen them since she got the news. Florence said, "Honestly, who could ask for more? I am so lucky."

In Florence's Own Words

"The very next day the kids surprised us and invited my sisters and brothers, and their spouses over to Guy & Janet's house. This would be the first time I'd seen them since I gave them my news. Guy, Janet, Clint and Vickie had prepared appetizers, and a really beautiful dinner for us. They waited on us and they ate in the kitchen while the rest of us ate in the dining room, so we could have the time with my sisters, brothers, and spouses. This is another thing I will never forget. It all meant so much to me. It was really wonderful. I just can't say enough about my son's and their wives, we are so much more than blessed. The things they do for us, its unbelievable."

Emails and Phone Calls

From the beginning, there was a steady flow of support and friendship, from family, members of our religious community, and then many friends, people whom I have worked with, people whose lives, joys, and sorrows I've shared in the past. As time went by, Florence would be inundated with emails. The emails were filled with optimism that everything would turn out fine and that Florence would do well. At least ninety-five percent of the emails received offered to say prayers for her.

I was deeply moved by the love that was pouring in from all over the country and Canada, and from as far away as Rome, Italy. We are so fortunate to have so many good and close friends.

One of the notes she received was from a wonderful Mormon family, friend's that go back some 50 years. Over the many years, Florence has come to be very close to the wife and mother of the family. This wonderful lady is truly the epitome of Mormon beliefs and the teachings of the Church of Latter Day Saints. I recall so many wonderful discussions with her and her husband, sharing both our faiths and belief systems. She writes,

"Nothing is ever hurt by prayer except the gates of hell. If we all take it to heart, we can turn this world toward God, once again. With God all things are possible. More importantly, how God hears and answers the prayers of the faithful. [1]*Give God thanks for the beautiful gift of your faith, for the powerful gift of prayer, and for the many miracles He works in your own daily life. Who says God does not work in mysterious ways? I asked the Lord to bless you as I prayed for you today. To guide you and protect you as you go along your way. His love is always with you; His promises are true, and when we give Him our cares you know He will see us through. So when the road you're traveling on seems difficult at best, just remember I'm here praying, and God will do the rest."*
- Love, Diane

From Ottawa, Canada, Florence received an email from Sr. Pauline Beauchesne, S.C.O., Sisters of Charity, the Grey Nuns of Montreal. Sr. Pauline told Florence that she continues to say daily prayers and offers her Mass for Florence from a chapel at the Motherhouse. Florence and

I first met Sr. Pauline on a trip to Ottawa to meet my mother's cousin, a retired nun at the Motherhouse.

In 2001, after my Mom passed away I was looking through old photos and letters written by my mom. One very old photo was a picture of my mom when she was three years old. She was sitting on the lap of her mother with her father standing next to her. There were other family members also in the photo. The photo was taken around 1916, and it was the only picture of mom's family, the Letourneau's. There was a cousin in the photo pictured near mom. Her name was Jean Letourneau who later took her vows, promising poverty, chastity and obedience as a Sister of Charity. Reading the old letters my mom wrote I found several addressed to Sister Jean. I was intrigued by the writings, which not only contained loving sentiments, but promises of baskets of Florida oranges that mom would send every year to the Motherhouse. I wanted very much to meet this lady, not only because she was family, but also to find out why mom was so immensely fond of her.

Arriving at the Sisters of Charity Motherhouse in Ottawa, Florence and I were greeted by Sr. Pauline who gave us a tour of the Motherhouse. The congregation of the Sisters of Charity of Ottawa was founded in 1845 by Elisabeth Bruyere whose name appears everywhere in the Ottawa Region. Towns, schools, churches, streets are named in her memory. After lunch, she took Florence and me to meet Sister Jean who had just turned 89. Why is it that nuns are always around five feet tall and have unblemished, beautiful faces? Sister Jean was a beautiful and wonderful person who Florence, and I fell in love with immediately. She spoke only French, and we spoke only English and yet we communicated with a little help from Sr. Pauline. We showed video films of my mom and dad and the photo where I first discovered Sr. Jean. Meeting her was one of my fondest moments and I will not forget her.

After our wonderful visit with Sr. Jean, Sr. Pauline took us to the chapel where Sr. Jean prayed everyday, the same chapel where today prayers are said on behalf of Florence. There is a closed circuit broadcast of the Mass coming from the chapel and into the lounge for the sisters living in the infirmary. Many of the sisters are too ill to make the trip upstairs to the chapel, but in the lounge the sisters can view and participate in the televised mass.

The women, all sporting snow-white hair, neat white habits and large silver crosses around their necks, watch as a priest holds up a chalice filled with wine. Many make their way to the lounge with their walkers, others with their wheelchairs. Some aren't able to get out of bed.

Most of the women like Sr. Jean were teenagers when they first walked the hallways of this same stone building. Young girls devoted to following in the footsteps of Elisabeth Bruyere as a Sister of Charity. Now, old and sick and after a lifetime of service, they have returned to the Motherhouse to find a peaceful refuge before they die. Now I understand why mom wrote so many times to Sr. Jean.

Sr. Jean Letourneau passed away peacefully at the Motherhouse of the Sisters of Charity, 9 Bruyere Street, at the age of ninety-nine, after sixty years of religious life.

Sr. Pauline and several friends continue to send their love and support. They have formed a common bond with Florence and their thoughtfulness has touched the both of us. We have saved all the emails and letters and will cherish them always.

Locating the Best Team of Doctors

Being diagnosed with cancer was traumatic for Florence. But now we needed to start the process of getting the best available doctors, the best information, and the best support from those we trusted. This would be one of the most important decisions we would be called on to make. We needed to find a team of specialists, surgeons, medical oncologists, and radiation oncologists. All of these doctors would be needed and would have to work together. This was a stressful time for us, yet it was so necessary to find the specialist we needed. After consulting with her primary care doctors, the names of a surgeon and an oncologist were given to us. The doctors told us that both of these physicians were very well regarded in the Orlando community and wanted us to at least talk to them. Things were moving very fast but in a positive way for Florence; and thanks to her primary care provider, the necessary appointments were scheduled.

I contacted my very good and close friend, Dr. Robert Baratta, a retired ophthalmologist and a true confidante. I've known Bob for over thirty-nine years and knew his opinions to be honest and forthright. He understood immediately my concerns about finding the right doctors for Florence and the importance of doing due diligence on those we would trust with Florence's health care. He offered to help get second opinions on her diagnosis and the biopsy results from doctors he knew who were well versed in breast cancer treatments.

Another physician, Dr. Jan Jablonski, was extraordinarily kind to Florence and me when she was made aware of Florence's condition. She is a long time friend. We watched her complete grade school, high school and finally graduated from medical school. Jan was aware of and knew many of the doctors in the local area and introduced us to the Florida Hospital Cancer Institute.

Our son Clint was also eager to be a part of the team. Clint had devoted many hours to the Leukemia and Lymphoma Society's Orlando chapter. As a participant in raising money for the Leukemia children (his heroes), he joined the Orlando Team in Training (TNT) group and participated in five Disney World marathons, three 100-mile bike rides and various other fund-raising events. Because of his association with the leukemia children, he had met some of the doctors who treated many of the children and was aware of the treatment programs available in our area.

Florence's chances for getting the best possible results were greatest when she was first diagnosed. We knew that the sooner we made decisions the greater her chances of a full recovery. But, we didn't want to rush into anything. Because of this, it was necessary that the specialists we would choose to be involved in her diagnosis, and potential treatments, would engage with us in discussions that would determine a strategy for the best cancer care for her. We gave the names of the oncologist and the surgeon to Clint and Jan to verify the qualifications of the doctors recommended by Florence's primary care physicians. They told us that Dr. Jon D. Wiese, the surgeon, and Dr. Sonalee K. Shroff, the Oncologist, were two of the very best in the Orlando area. Both had excellent reputations and a knowledgebase of experience in breast cancer. Dr. Shroff practices her skills at the Florida Hospital Cancer Institute in Orlando, Florida where Florence would spend a lot of time. The Florida Hospital Cancer Institute serves more cancer patients than any other healthcare system in Florida, and also enjoys a fine reputation in cancer research and technology.

Finding doctors who were board-certified and had training in breast cancer treatment was important to us. Even though board certification does not exist for breast cancer surgery, a board-certified doctor in general surgery would provide the essential skills needed to treat Florence and potentially perform breast surgery on her. Dr. Wiese was board certified and had performed breast cancer surgery for many years and certainly was qualified and experienced.

We needed doctors who would fight for Florence, no matter how big the challenge, and who would not be intimidated by how grave her illness might be. We wanted them to fight with all the vigor, skills, and techniques that they could muster. Dr. Wiese and Dr. Shroff were those kind of doctors. We felt that they would give us the best chance to defeat her cancer.

If Florence was to have surgery, and that was becoming a very real possibility, there would be a protocol of treatments after surgery, which would include not only a medical oncologist, but also a radiologist.

The radiologist uses radiation after a lumpectomy or mastectomy is performed. Since breast tissue is extremely sensitive to damage by radiation, it is crucial to find competent and experienced practitioners who have at their disposal the best equipment possible for the delivery of radiation treatment. Dr. Wiese and Dr. Shroff both recommended Dr. David A. Diamond, a Radiation Oncologist who was a staff member at the Florida Hospital Cancer Institute. Again, Jan and Clint were there for us and found his credentials, his experience and his expertise in cancer treatments the best in the community.

When Florence was told she had breast cancer it was extremely upsetting. It was as if her world had turned upside down. But it was necessary now, to take the time, to talk to our closest friends and family, and to compose our selves. We were not going to be urged by any doctor to move ahead without understanding what was happening. A good physician should encourage us to ask questions and he or she should be thoughtful and understandable. We asked them to carefully explain to us, all the available options in Florence's treatment and their feelings about them. If they used any medical or technical terms that were not familiar to us, we asked them for a layperson's translation.

It was starting to be clear to us that we were indeed fortunate to have the Florida Hospital Cancer Institute team of medical oncologists, radiation oncologists, surgeons, and other specialists providing us the best team of physicians; and they were right here in Orlando, Florida. But who will be in charge of this team? That was easy Florence would be in charge! She would need to work with the team that will be giving her the best treatment program available. Each member having skill sets for each of the required specialty. It will be essential that she feel comfortable with all of the doctors who will be responsible for her care, and equally important that she be convinced that the treatment suggested is best for her. She will become the leader of the team! She knows the treatment of breast cancer will be a cooperative effort, but at all times this is about her. She is the patient - in charge!

The Biopsy Results

Our first meeting with our surgeon, Dr. Wiese, was on Tuesday, July 10th. The lump was malignant, and Florence was facing surgery to remove the tumor. The news caused feelings of disbelief and denial that this could be happening to her. It was a most distressing and difficult situation for the both of us to listen to the doctor's explanation of the results. Florence was in tears even though she had known that this was a real possibility. But now the news was official, and somehow it felt her world had just collapsed. The doctor gave us a moment or two to compose ourselves. There was nothing I could say but just hold her, console her, and let her feel my love for her. It was again, another moment of intense feelings I had for her, and there would be many more to come.

Florence had been diagnosed with Ductal Carcinoma, which could be at a stage two or three. Florence's tumor was poorly differentiated and estrogen/progesterone positive, which in the past was considered a poor prognosis. You accept the truth, as hard as it may be. But somewhere, deep down, we felt an urge to fight this cancer with everything we had. We weren't going to be frustrated and overwhelmed by this beast.

The surgeon discussed the findings thus far, and told Florence she had options as to what type of surgery would be available to her. At that time, we knew nothing about breast cancer let alone what her treatment outcome would be so we were scared. We were bombarded with information about her tumor size, cancer type, whether her lymph nodes were involved, and many other topics. Just about every time Florence was to make a decision, she had two more choices. There was no right answer. Her decisions were based not only on the nature of her tumor, but also her doctor's advice. She had to make decisions despite being emotional, vulnerable, and upset with the diagnosis that she had cancer.

Florence has cancer; cancer doesn't have Florence. I also believe that the comment about people going through the various stages of coping with cancer differently is very true. My experience was a feeling of frustration, grief, and finally acceptance. Now it was time to get on with the battle we now faced. I knew the burden of breast cancer fell on Florence, and I knew that I would have to be the caretaker knowing full well my ineptitude - "I can't even remember when I last did the laundry or cooked an egg." I needed to learn quickly; after all, my wife would be fighting a life-threatening disease. I needed to be on top of everything. I needed to be there for her and to listen to what she was saying. I needed to help figure out what to do, especially when she may be too shocked and anguished to take everything in the doctors were saying to her.

In Florence's Own Words

"Met with my surgeon Dr. Jon Wiese. I was very nervous since this whole thing had been so scary since I got this news, and I'm now meeting the guy who will do the surgery. As soon as he walked in the door, I had a feeling of comfort come over me. The more we talked, the more I felt very safe about him and when I left I felt very happy he would be the one. The thing that really impressed me was when he was talking to me I started to get emotional and I didn't want Guy to see me cry (he was sitting behind me). Dr. Wiese picked up on this and just kept talking giving me time to gain my composure. I really appreciated that."

Lumpectomy or Mastectomy

Florence had a choice between a lumpectomy and a mastectomy. This was not a life or death decision, but it was a significant decision. Florence said with as much courage as she could muster, "Doctor, give me your best recommendation as to what I should do? I don't care if you have to remove one or both breasts; I want this thing out of my body!"

The doctor went on to explain, the lumpectomy patients have a forty percent chance of a local recurrence, another cancer in the same breast, unless they have radiation following their surgery. With a lumpectomy plus radiation, the patient has about a ten percent chance of local recurrence for invasive cancer. Florence was a good candidate for lumpectomy surgery (a partial mastectomy), and it is a less severe surgery. In addition, the surgeon told us that a lumpectomy followed by radiation treatments yields a rate of local recurrence, in the breast itself, only few percentage points higher than the rate for the mastectomy patient.

My mind was working overtime. Isn't it ironic that in the USA breasts are highly regarded and a very big deal with women? I didn't care if Florence had two, three or none; I was very much in love with her. Her breasts or lack there of, was not going to change who she was or what I thought of her.

I said to her, "What do you think, Sweetheart, lumpectomy sure sounds good to me," as I held back the tears. Florence took a deep breath and said. "Lumpectomy surgery sounds good to me."

Florence's scheduled meeting with Dr. Sonalee K. Shroff, her oncologist at the Florida Hospital Cancer Institute, was to discuss the post-surgery treatment options that would be available to her. When Florence started to walk in, she looked up and saw the sign on the building that read, Florida Cancer Institute. Later Florence said to me, "I couldn't believe I was going there for me. It took my breath away." But, she took a step forward, a deep breath and walked in. That moment in time, the sign, the word cancer everywhere, was a defining moment in our lives. This was real. It was happening! Nothing was going to change! Keep on going and don't give up. We will not let cancer control us

In Florence's Own Words

"Thursday I had an appointment with my oncologist and Guy dropped me off in front of the door and he went to park. When I started to walk in, I looked up and saw "Florida Cancer Institute", it felt like someone punched me, I couldn't believe I was going in there for me. But, I took a step forward, a deep breath, walked in and I was fine, not really, but I had to move on. So I'm sure there will be those times where I'll just need to focus on family and friends and know their prayers and thoughts are there for me."

Sleep Loss

Sleeping at night had not been a problem for me until Florence was diagnosed. Now, I'm an extremely light sleeper and wake frequently throughout the night. I knew my inability to sleep had to do with the constant stress I was under with what seemed to be a roller coaster of decisions that needed to be made daily. Tossing and turning all night long had made me miserable and was not without consequences. I was tense and scared, under pressure, watching Florence as she faced all of the medical treatments and tests she had to go through. These anxiety attacks, although a natural response, were aggravating and were the biggest reasons I could not sleep. Inadvertent weight loss was just one example of how to much stress and the loss of sleep affected me. Within a couple of months, I was down from 228 to 214 pounds. It seems the hardest places stress hits us are in our bedrooms and in our stomachs. I also know if I don't get enough sleep I won't be able to remove myself from this current stress in my life.

Someone suggested keeping a journal, writing down everything Flo and I do daily. Doing this organizes what happens daily and allows my brain to focus on the day's events. Surprisingly, I have been keeping a diary. The diary was in the form of emails. Since Florence was first diagnosed I have written, and archived chronologically, emails to my family and friends, including all of their responses. However, the one thing more fulfilling than keeping these emails was reading them, especially the responses. As it turns out, this activity of keeping a diary (email diary) has turned out to be like my own personal psychiatrist and has been the primary source of the content of this book. It has lessened my anxiety and stress significantly, and I'm able to sleep much better – at least most of the time.

Stress is a part of our modern society. I found in research that, "if people didn't suffer any stress at all, nothing would get done, and if people suffer too much stress it could be harmful to the mind and body." People work long hours, worry about the future, forgo sleep and get caught up in the rat race, rather than take the time for meditation and reflection. As for me, I was so fortunate to have found the St. Stephen Chapel where I could meditate and reflect on what was going on around me. And, as I said before, it was the "quiet zone" I very much needed - my stress reliever.

The Crane

Florence and I entered the Cancer Institute and asked the information attendant for directions to Dr. Shroff's office. "Elevator to your left, 3rd floor, take a right, room 381." That was easy; we thought a little quick but easy. We entered the elevator, pushed the third floor button and waited for the door to open. The elevator came to a stop, and the door opened. As we walked out, we stopped immediately. In the front of us was a beautiful painting of a crane hanging on the wall. We stared for a minute or two at the painting. Within those seconds, we both felt a deep feeling of comfort that this meeting with Dr. Shroff would be very positive for Florence. In many parts of the world cranes are revered as the messengers of peace. Cranes are symbols of happiness, beauty, and love. They are killers of snakes and so, in Christian symbolism, the enemies of the devil.

Our family has a history of wonderful stories of the crane. When looking back at those stories, they seem to be derived from a period of depression after losing a loved one or perhaps, a reminder of a sad time in our life. I remember the week shortly after the funeral of my sister-in-law. I had just finished jogging and was sitting outside on the pool deck drinking a cup of coffee when a beautiful white bird landed on the patio only ten feet from me. I was startled by its presence, and how close it was to me. I slowly turned from the table staring, wondering if it would fly away. Yes, it was a crane. I was told later that the closest a white bird had come to the house was near the boat dock some two hundred feet away. They never had a bird this large land on the patio this close. Numerous times after that day members of our family, close to my sister-in-Law, had similar encounters with a crane in other odd places and would be reminded of the sad week when she died.

I have always been skeptical hearing about things like cranes appearing for no reason, or even stories of spiritual apparitions were difficult for me to comprehend and believe. I'm laughing at myself as I'm writing this - comparing religious apparitions with cranes. Yet, there was a side of me that was extremely envious of those whose faith was so much stronger than mine. They believe not only in their religion and its teachings but also in religious apparitions. Many believed that birds, like the crane, could be messengers from heaven.

Having a large bird land next to me was indeed an awakening experience, especially during the events of that week with all the preparation for the funeral going on around me. Yet, it was difficult for me to make a connection with the passing of a loved one, and the visit of this majestic bird, the crane. It took a second visit for me to think twice of why this bird appears and continues to appear at times when there is difficulty in our lives.

Recently, Florence and I had the opportunity to take care of my mother and father during the last phases of their lives. My mom was battling cancer and my dad struggled with Parkinson's. After we received the news that my Mom had only six months to live, we moved my dad to a nursing home.

I had taken Mom to a scheduled meeting with her oncologist to receive an assessment on her condition and chemotherapy treatments. I remember asking her doctor if the treatments were working. She said, "I'm afraid not, Guy."

I looked at my Mom; she stared back at me, with a smile, not saying anything. I thought to myself, what does that mean? "Doctor," I said, "what are we talking about? How much time?" The doctor answered, "Six months, maybe. You never really know, but I think around six months or so."

I was astonished at Mom's reaction and finally, her question. "So, doctor," she said with a smile, "I'm on borrowed time, aren't I?" The doctor looked at me, and we stared at her with a smile. I was thinking, and I'm sure the doctor was too, what a wonderful lady to simultaneously grasp and accept the severity of this news.

"Yes Mom," whispering to myself, "you are on borrowed time."

Mom died exactly six months later on June 24th. It was during the week of preparing for Mom's Memorial Mass when I found myself in the garage doing some cleanup. The garage door was open behind me when I felt someone staring. Many have had that feeling, someone behind staring. You don't want to turn around, yet you have to. I slowly turned around and looking through the garage door opening I saw a large white crane on the sidewalk. We both stared at each other as it slowly walked up the driveway to the entrance of the garage. I didn't move. I just stared at it. I was wondering would it come into the garage? It stopped at the entrance for a moment, never taking its eyes off me. I was amazed how brave it was to be this close to a human, let alone at the doorway of the garage. It just continued to stare. I'm thinking to myself, how can I get Florence's attention without scaring it away? I want her to see this so badly, yet I can't yell for her. I simply whispered to the bird, "Hello." I can't believe I just said that. I'm talking to a bird. Less than a minute later, or so, the crane turned around, walked down the driveway, made a left onto the sidewalk, and continued walking past our neighbors homes and then flew away. I immediately called Florence to come out to the garage where I described the whole event to her; except, I didn't tell her that I said hello to the bird. By the way, there is no water source as one might expect cranes and other aquatic birds to be near. We have never seen a crane in this neighborhood since we lived here, so why this visit? Not sure! I would say it was a stressful time during the week, and I just received a message from heaven – maybe even from Mom.

Having a crane appear, always gave this family a sense of remembrance, a sense that our loved ones who have gone before us were watching out for each of us. Human spirit is resilient, and somehow you will find the strength to carry on. Perhaps the crane reminds us of that spirit.

Throughout history, birds have been seen as animals of unique value and have meanings from legends and stories that have survived over generations. [2]In Japanese, Chinese, and Korean tradition, cranes stand for good fortune and longevity because of its fabled life span of a thousand years. The Japanese refers to the crane as "the bird of happiness." [3]The Chinese refer them as "heavenly cranes," believing they were symbols of wisdom. The powerful wings of the crane were believed to be able to convey souls up to paradise and to take people to higher levels of spiritual enlightenment.

After my encounter with the crane, I read this wonderful Japanese legend of a young girl, Sadako Sasaki from Hiroshima.

According to a [2]Japanese legend, the crane lives for a thousand years, and a sick person who folds 1,000 origami cranes ("Origami" is the ancient Japanese art of paper folding) will become well again. [4]A young girl, Sadako Sasaki from Hiroshima, set out to do just that when she developed leukemia as a result of her exposure to the atomic bomb dropped on her city. She died at age twelve before her project was completed. [5]Her classmates folded the remaining cranes for Sadako after her death and placed them at the foot of a monument constructed in Sadako's memory in Hiroshima's National Peace Park. The statue depicts Sadako holding a golden crane in her arms. At the base of the statue a plaque reads, "This is our cry, this is our prayer, peace in the world." Each year, on August 6, thousands of origami cranes from all over the world are placed beneath Sadako's statue.

Herceptin

Florence and I were pleased by Dr. Shroff's candor and expertise. Florence felt confident in her explanation of the different treatment programs and knew she would be in good hands. Dr. Shroff told us there is a new marker for the Her-2/neu, and there is a particular treatment for cancer cells that have over expression of this protein. The new drug is Herceptin (her-SEP-tin) and some oncologists want to give it to patients before their surgery to shrink the tumor. Florence's decision will be, does she shrink the tumor first with Herceptin, or go with the surgery first. We talked about the new treatment protocols available and considered some chemo recipes that would include Herceptin.

Herceptin is a treatment for women with breast cancer whose tumors have too much HER2 protein. This type of cancer is known as HER2-positive, HER2/neu, or HER2 over expressing. HER2/neu tumors tend to grow and spread more quickly than tumors that are not HER2/neu. This is why it is so important to find out Florence's cancer HER2 status. Clinical experience with Herceptin for the adjuvant treatment of HER2/neu, node-positive breast cancers, began in 2000. In 2006, Herceptin was approved for the adjuvant treatment of HER2/neu, node-positive breast cancer. This was a new medication and I was told it was the newest and latest in cancer treatment protocols. Herceptin is not chemotherapy or hormonal therapy. Herceptin is a type of targeted cancer treatment known as targeted biologic therapy. Antibodies are part of the body's normal defense against bacteria, viruses, and abnormal cells, such as cancer cells. Herceptin is designed to target HER2/neu cancer cells. It works by attaching itself to a HER2/neu cancer cell and tells the body's defense system to target the HER2/neu cancer cell. It also stops the HER2/neu cancer cell from telling itself to grow and divide into more cancer cells.

Ok, now I need to get technical; actually it's interesting how this technology works. I think it's important you stay with me through these next segments.

Herceptin blocks the estrogen receptor. Estrogen comes in and attaches to a receptor that sends a message to the nucleus that tells the cell to grow. Here is the good part. Herceptin comes into the receptor and it blocks it so that the natural estrogen cannot get into the receptor. Does this remind you of a lock and key analogy? It's the key that goes into the lock and gets stuck. It doesn't turn the lock open and, therefore, it cannot send the cell the message to divide.

What exactly is HER2? HER2 stands for Human Epidermal growth factor Receptor 2. Each healthy breast cell includes copies of the HER2 gene, which helps healthy cells grow. The HER2 gene is found in the DNA of a cell, and this gene contains the information for making the HER2 protein. The HER2 protein, also called the HER2 receptor, is found on the surface of some healthy cells in the body. In normal cells, HER2 proteins help send growth signals from outside the cell to the inside of the cell. These signals tell the cell to grow and divide.

In Florence's HER2/neu breast cancer, the cancer cells have an abnormally high number of HER2 genes per cell. When this happens, too many HER2 proteins, appears on the surface of these cancer cells. This is called HER2 protein over expression. Too many HER2 protein is believe to cause cancer cells to grow and divide more quickly. This is why HER2/neu breast cancer is often more aggressive than breast cancer that is not HER2/neu, and this is the reasoning for adding Herceptin as part of Florence's treatment protocol.

Vascular Port Implant

Dr. Shroff recommended that Florence take Herceptin weekly for fifty-two weeks. Once Florence starts Herceptin, she will also receive other chemotherapy drugs for the first eighteen weeks of Herceptin therapy. After completion of the chemotherapy, Herceptin will be given on its own. Clinical trial results showed that Herceptin, in addition to chemotherapy reduced the risk of cancer returning by fifty-two percent compared to chemotherapy alone. The question was what combination of chemotherapy drugs would be added along with the Herceptin. Dr. Shroff suggested two drugs, Taxotere and Carboplatin, though she could not be sure until the tumor could be analyzed in more detail after Florence's surgery.

Dr. Shroff also suggested prior to chemotherapy, the installation of a central venous access port device in Florence's chest to facilitate the administration of all of the drugs. Intravenous access would be easier for Florence using a port than finding a vein each time. Unlike typical catheters, which exit from the skin, this catheter will be inserted by tunneling under the skin into the internal jugular vein. The other end of the catheter will interface with the port that is placed completely below the skin. With a port, a raised disk is felt underneath the skin. Blood is drawn or medication delivered by placing a needle through the overlying skin into the port or reservoir. These devices have greatly improved infusion access for cancer patients. They have reduced the risk of medication infusion problems such as phlebitis and tissue damage. Additionally the added bonus has been the ability to draw blood through them for routine laboratory tests.

Unfortunately, along with all the many benefits, complications may still occur. The diagnosis of cancer and potential treatments for this disease may put patients at higher risk for complications associated with the use of a vascular access device. These can include blood clots, and nearby vein infections. Patients have an added risk of increased infections due to their suppressed immune system. There is also the possibility of inaccurate lab test results due to loss of integrity of the blood vessel or poor circulation in the area of the port. The frequency of these complications is directly related to how often the port is used.

In spite of potential complications, Florence wanted her surgeon, Dr. Wiese, to perform the procedure of placing the vascular access device in her chest, above her right breast. I called him and scheduled a surgery date a few days before Florence would start her chemotherapy treatments.

We ended our visit with Dr. Shroff with Florence feeling very good about the answers to the many questions we asked. It would be important for Florence to make the commitment to follow Dr. Shroff's recommended treatment plans as soon as she recovers from her lumpectomy surgery, but now it was time to schedule a regimen of tests that would tell us if the cancer did or did not invade other organs or parts of her body. During the next week and a half, Florence would be tested using state-of-the-art technology: CT scans, PET scans, Bone and MUGA scans.

Florence had done the single most difficult thing to begin her journey - she made a commitment to do whatever it took to beat this cancer. She started by getting the best possible medical team, doing everything she could, and leaving nothing out that might be of help to her. Now it was time for her to complete her commitment. Everyone says a positive mental attitude is an important ingredient when fighting cancer, but it is not a simple matter of thinking positive. It is a matter of knowledge. Knowledge is power! It is a matter of educating ourselves about every detail and mustering every resource available to us.

In Florence's Own Words

"Had Port Implant for upcoming chemo treatments. Very apprehensive the past few days! Had a few anxiety attacks and scared (I know that's all anticipation/fear of not knowing.) But everything turned out fine. The only thing I felt was when I ate dinner. I could feel the tube as I chewed and it felt weird, and it seemed to roll a little, that's all. I only took one pain pill and slept well. Dr. Wiese was great and also made me feel comfortable about all of this.

Guy has been glued to my side since all of this started. I sure hope that glue continues to stick, because I would become very unglued if it doesn't. I love him!!!"

Learning About Cancer

The process of trying to learn about cancer was difficult. I never attended medical school, or studied other related subjects. Florence and I once visited a Body Worlds exhibition in Phoenix. During the visit I learned about Plastination, a new technique for odorless preservation of cadavers and about anatomic structure and function of our bodies. That's the extent of my medical knowledge. Now I needed to educate myself about the world of cancer and especially, breast cancer. I was somewhat surprised at the extent of material, documentation, and vast amounts of data, good and bad that was available. On the Internet all I had to do is type the word cancer in a search engine and I was inundated with material. Eventually I found what I was looking for... what is cancer? Here is a short synopsis of what I found.

[6]If cells divide when new cells are not needed, they form too much tissue. The mass or lump of extra tissue, called a tumor, can be benign or malignant. Malignant tumors are cancer. The cancer cells grow and divide out of control; they also become undifferentiated, which means they lose the distinguishing characteristic of the original tissue. [7]They can invade and damage nearby tissues and organs. Also, cancer cells can break away from a malignant tumor and enter the bloodstream or lymphatic system. That is how breast cancer spreads and forms secondary tumors in other parts of the body. The spread of cancer is called metastasis.

I continued to search out anything and everything that related to Florence's cancer, her treatment and all the tests she would have to go through. My breast cancer binder was getting filled quickly with documentation on all aspects of her cancer, lumpectomy, chemotherapy, radiation, and the various drugs she would take.

From the research, I found that one hundred years ago one in thirty-three people were diagnosed with cancer. Cancer was a mysterious disease few understood, and even fewer survived it. Today in the United States, one woman is diagnosed with breast cancer every three minutes, and one woman will die of breast cancer every thirteen minutes. Even though these are alarming statistics, a woman's five-year survival rate is above ninety-seven percent in cases in which the breast cancer is detected early.

Breast cancer is undeniably difficult, but it will not define Florence. She will remain the same wonderful and unique person I have always known and loved. She may be a cancer patient, but she is not a cancer victim.

Ten Days of Tests

Florence's medical testing will not only be an important component but will be an unavoidable part of her journey. All of the test procedures are designed to monitor the progression and/or remission of the disease. It will also measure the success or failure of the treatment she's about to undergo. Her oncologist will make use of all of the information gathered from the tests to guide her in making proper recommendations to us. But every test, difficult or not, will again evoke all of the anxieties while waiting for the results. The usual routine seen every day in a doctor's office or laboratory is far different from our new routine since the results will alter the course of Florence's life. Florence will be giving up a year of her life fighting this insidious disease. A sacrifice she will make in the interest of the rest of her life. Her spirit is resilient, and somehow - somehow, she will find the strength to carry on.

Florence's first test was a PET scan that helped the doctor effectively pinpoint the source of her cancer. [8]This is possible because many cancer cells are highly metabolic and, therefore, synthesize the radioactive glucose (sugar) that was injected in Florence prior to the scan. The areas of high glucose are displayed as bright areas on the PET scan. Florence's entire body was scanned to identify whether cancer was isolated to one particular area or had spread to other organs.

The next test Florence took was a computed tomography scan, otherwise called a CT scan. The CT scan uses X-rays to produce detailed pictures of structures inside the body. During the test, Florence lay on a table that was attached to the CT scanner, a large doughnut-shaped machine. The CT scanner sends X-rays through the body areas being studied. An iodine dye used as a contrast material is used to create structures and organs easier to see on the CT images. The dye is used to find tumors, and look for other problems.

The injection of the dye was very difficult for Florence. Since her earlier biopsy procedure was on her left breast, they used her right arm to find a vein for the IV. Locating adequate veins for an IV has always been difficult for Florence. Sometimes they even had to place the IV on the top of her hand. This was very painful for her, and I always had to turn away.

There are ever-present concerns when one is taking chemotherapy that there will be adverse side effects. Some chemotherapeutic agents can be quite toxic to the heart muscle. Herceptin, in particular, may cause heart issues, and since it was to be prescribed by Dr. Shroff, it would be necessary to assess the function of Florence's heart. Doing an MUGA scan does this. MUGA is an acronym for Multiple Gated Acquisition. By measuring Florence's heart functions periodically during chemotherapy, Dr. Shroff can determine, on an ongoing basis, whether it is safe to continue with the therapy, or whether certain medications need to be stopped.

Dr. Shroff had also ordered a FISH (Fluorescence in-situ hybridization) test to determine whether Florence had HER2-positive breast cancer. This analysis can be made at the same time as her initial breast cancer surgery. Samples of her cancer tissue from previous biopsies or surgery may be used. FISH testing measures the amount of the HER2/neu gene in each cell. This gene is responsible for the overproduction of the HER2 protein. There is no number scale for FISH testing. The result is either: FISH-negative, a standard number of the genes is present, or FISH-positive; an excessive number of the genes is present. This is sometimes called gene amplification. A cancer with too many of these genes is called HER2-positive. [9]If a cancer is HER2-positive, it may respond to Herceptin. Herceptin, remember, is the drug that can slow down or stop the growth of cancer with too many HER2 genes.

Florence's Courage

After completing a bone scan, her last test, we were walking down the hallway toward the exit of the Cancer Research Hospital. Florence said, "Boy that was really tough! It was so painful when they injected the contrast in me. The whole time I kept thinking about Clint and his heroes." Florence was referring to the children who struggle everyday with Leukemia and have to be injected with chemo drugs. "If those children can put up with the needles, so can I. I have nothing to complain about."

I was so overwhelmed with what she said, that I purposely slowed down to walk behind her and hide the emotions building up inside me. I did not want her to see me lose it. I tried hard to stay focused, looking away from her, and toward the wall. There were beautiful paintings hanging on the wall, paintings of cancer survivors, each one with wonderful messages of hope. I pointed to one, making sure she would not see my face, and said, "Florence, look at that painting on the wall." The message on the painting said, "I believe life is a journey and my destination will be blessed."

Some of the other paintings we looked at had the following messages:

"I believe God carries my heart"
"I believe in faith and family"
"I believe in the healing power of prayer"
"I believe in God, family and friends"
"I believe I have more to do"

After composing myself, and hoping she had not seen my face, we continued walking, holding each other's hands, not saying anything. It was the statement about the leukemia heroes that opened my eyes and told me more about her character; a character trait she always had, but I never really understood. I knew she was strong, but I never realized the depth of her strength.

This was a woman who will soon experience, courageously, - pain, fear, sorrow, and joy. I so much admire her strength. She is a hero to me, to her loved ones, and I believe a hero to God.

We will know the outcome of the tests at a doctor's visit on July 31st. Again we have to deal with the anxiety that comes from waiting, not knowing what the results will be or how the lumpectomy surgery will go. There really isn't anything we can do about waiting except to hope and pray that the people we have on our team will come through for us. It's a feeling of helplessness. Florence will be facing the surgeon's knife, the oncologist's recipe of chemicals, and then the radiation, not to mention all of the unforeseen complications and side effects that were likely to appear. What is chemotherapy? What are its side effects really like? How will radiation affect Florence? She is now living with a life-threatening illness that may return or worsen at any time.

Test Results - The Prayers are working

On July 31st, we met with Dr. Shroff to discuss the results of a week and a half of testing. My brave lady endured being poked in the hand and arm with needles that were inserted into her veins. She was injected with radioactive glucose, radioactive isotopes, and radionuclide. It was the equivalent of over two hundred normal X-rays. She was placed into small holes and tunnels in the center of large machines, trying hard not to become claustrophobic. She finally completed the entire test series, and now we were ready to hear the results.

Holding our breath, Florence and I listened patiently to Dr. Shroff as she looked at the PET, CT, Bone and MUGA tests. She said, "From what I am reading here, all of your tests seem to be normal. It doesn't look like the cancer has spread, and it is probably localized in your breast. The CT scan shows a small spot around L3, lower back, but it's probably calcium, a little arthritis maybe, not to worry, we'll do an MRI and check it out."

The good news is Florence's PET, CAT and Bone scan showed no indication that the cancer had spread into her Lymph nodes. However, we will only know during and after her surgery, if this is indeed accurate. The FISH test confirmed her Biopsy as being positive for a Hercep2 positive tumor. We expected that, so it wasn't a surprise. The cancer is an aggressive form, but it seems to be contained.

The news was indeed good for Florence. It gave her so much more confidence that she would beat this intrusion of an unwanted invader into her body. However, we were cautious not to be overexcited, as we both knew it would still be a long and difficult road for Florence to travel.

The following day we met with her surgeon, Dr. Wiese, who confirmed the test results. Again we discussed the merits of lumpectomy versus mastectomy. And again, with the help of Dr. Wiese, Florence chose the lumpectomy procedure. I asked what the procedure entails and what can Florence expect after the surgery. I was told that basically, it is a three-part procedure. First, a Sentinel Lymph Node Biopsy is performed; second, they mark and target the exact location of the tumor, and third, the actual removal of the tumor. After her surgery, Florence will be taken to a recovery room. She will stay there until she is awake and her condition and vital signs (blood pressure, pulse, breathing, etc.) are stable. The operation would take approximately two to three hours, and if there were no complications, she would be able to come home that evening. "What about drains?" I asked. Dr. Wiese replied, "Its possible Florence may have one or more drains, depending on the extent of the surgical procedure." What he was telling us made me feel apprehensive and uneasy. I had read extensive articles on breast cancer surgery and understood that doctors really don't know the full extent of the cancer until they peel back layers of tissue and determine, with the help of a pathologist, the nature of the tumor. If the lymph nodes are involved then the surgeon will perform a lymph node dissection. He may remove some or all of the lymph nodes under her arm. The drains, rubber tubes coming out from the breast or underarm area, are there to remove blood and lymph fluid that collects during the healing process. Most drains stay in place for one or two weeks. When drainage has decreased to about 30 cc, 1 fluid ounce, each day, the drains can be removed. As a general rule, women having lymph node dissection stay in the hospital for one or two nights and then go home. If she does come home the same day, we may need a home care nurse to monitor and provide care.

The possibility exists that, during the surgery, the surgeon may find that the cancer was more extensive than was first diagnosed. If so, a mastectomy would be required. Florence would have to come back at a later date for the mastectomy surgery. The reason the doctor cannot perform the mastectomy right then is because it is a completely different procedure and requires permission from our insurance company.

Listening to Dr. Wiese, and trying to comprehend everything, I was starting to feel overwhelmed. "Too much information," I thought to myself. Perhaps I was trying too hard to be clinical and not understanding the material I was reading.

Dr. Wiese was very kind to Florence and me as he explained the procedure. Florence later would say, "I am blessed to be so comfortable with him. When he talks to me, I feel safe. He has such a calming effect on me, and I really think I'm in good hands with him."

The three of us agreed to Wednesday, August 13th as the date to remove the tumor. Again, the waiting starts, the anxieties set in. In twelve days, one of the most important events in Florence's life will take place.

Florence and I began getting hints about the upcoming chemo protocol after her surgery. She and I began to understand the difficulties she would be facing. The good news was we were involved with the latest protocols available and would continue to have discussions with her oncologist as to the best treatment for her. I was somewhat excited and cautiously optimistic about the treatment aimed at removing this beast from her body. But more than that, we would have the opportunity to have other opinions as to the best approach.

In Florence's Own Words

"Visited Dr. Shroff for test results and protocol. All tests came back with no other problems. Protocol will be: Three chemicals (including Herceptin) once every 3 weeks for 18 weeks. Approximately 2/3 weeks after that will get radiation everyday except weekends for 6 and a half weeks. Herceptin (cancer preventative) will continue every week for a year. UGH!!!"

Being a Caretaker

As I mentioned earlier, fighting cancer is not a simple matter of thinking positively, although necessary, it really is a matter of knowledge. I need to educate myself about every detail. I need to stop fearing cancer and start taking a proactive role. I will go to every appointment. I need to be there for Florence. I will be glued to her hip, and in that way, I will contribute to Florence's battle. I will be her caretaker, her partner.

As an official breast cancer husband and caretaker, I join a very unique group of husbands who have to walk the walk and talk the talk for the sake of their spouses. Men, who have in their own ways contributed so much to their wives' welfare, and husbands who have changed their lifestyles and given of themselves to take care of that special person in their lives. These guys are the ones for whom I have such admiration. They've been there they've done that.

With all the anxiety and depression triggered by Florence's diagnoses; and now with the stress of the pending surgery and treatments, Florence will need the emotional and physical support I know I can give her. I want to be as good as all of the other caretakers out there. Love is everything here, and we will need the support of our family: our two sons, our daughters-in-law, and our grandchildren. Also, I know that Florence will do so much better in the long run with the love of her brothers and sisters. My job will be to give that extra snuggle, hold her hand, and most of all, say the "I love you." All of this will make the difference during her down time. My information file is already growing, and the goal will be to acquire all the necessary information that will allow me to ask the intelligent questions each time we visit the doctors. There's no way we will become victims to this insidious disease.

The words of Vince Lombardi,

"It's not whether you get knocked down, it's whether you get back up,"

These words resonate in my mind.

August 13th - Time For Surgery

After arriving at the hospital, Florence proceeded to check in, signing all of the necessary disclaimers and approvals. After the paperwork ritual, we were asked to go to pre-op for the first procedure before surgery. There would be three procedures that Florence would go through. The first procedure is called a Sentinel Lymph Node Biopsy. The former tests Florence had gone through indicated her lymph nodes were not involved. But the doctors wouldn't really know for sure until the surgery. The "Sentinel Lymph Node" is the first node to which the cancer cells are likely to spread from Florence's tumor. This procedure will be used to help determine the extent, or stage, of Florence's cancer. It also allows the surgeon the opportunity to decide a better plan for the operation, if necessary.

The procedure identifies where the sentinel lymph node is located. Injecting a radioactive substance does this or blue dye, or both near the tumor. The surgeon then uses a scanner to find the lymph node containing the radioactive substance, or looks for the lymph node stained with dye. This is the sentinel node. The surgeon will then make a small incision in the skin overlying the sentinel lymph node and remove it.

A pathologist checks the sentinel node under a microscope for the presence of cancer cells. [10]If cancer is found, the surgeon will usually remove more lymph nodes during the biopsy procedure or during a follow-up surgical procedure.

What are the benefits for Florence of going through this procedure? First, one needs to understand standard lymph node removal. [10]Standard lymph node removal involves surgery to remove most of the lymph nodes in the area of the tumor. These are called regional lymph nodes. For example, breast cancer surgery may include removing most of the auxiliary lymph nodes, [10]the group of lymph nodes under the arm. This is called auxiliary lymph node dissection.

If sentinel lymph node biopsy is done and the sentinel node does not contain cancer cells, the rest of the regional lymph nodes may not need to be removed. Because fewer lymph nodes are removed, there would be fewer side effects. [10]When multiple regional lymph nodes are removed, the patient may experience side effects such as lymphedema, a swelling caused by excess fluid build-up. There are other potential side effects such as numbness, a persistent burning sensation, infection, and difficulty moving the affected body area.

The second procedure involved needle wires being inserted by a radiologist to target the tumor. Wire localization is used for markers showing optimal excision margins for the surgeon so that he will be more precise as he performs the lumpectomy. After numbing the area with a local anesthetic, a hollow needle, thinner than that used for drawing blood, is placed into the breast, and x-rays are used to guide the needle to the suspicious area. A thin wire is then inserted through the center of the needle. A small hook at the end of the wire keeps it in place. The hollow needle is then removed. The surgeon will use the wires as a guide to locate the abnormal areas to be removed.

After the first two procedures, the hospital tech brought the two of us into a small cubicle with curtains around it. Florence was asked to take off her clothes and put on a hospital gown and slippers. She lay back on the hospital bed and rested. The technician started to prep her for surgery installing an IV for hydration, anesthesia, and other drugs that may be needed in the operation. Again, and as before, Florence's veins were small and difficult to tap into, and this caused her pain. The nurse was very attentive to the problem and used a butterfly needle, which was smaller than a regular needle. Watching carefully all of the procedures, I wanted to connect with her in a physical way but wasn't sure how. The truth is I wanted to trade positions with her and take the pain myself. Instead, I sat silently in a chair by her side. We both looked at each other, and a small smile appeared across her worried face. I reached out and we held hands as we waited for the next step.

In Florence's Own Words

"Big Day!! Lumpectomy. I just can't believe this is happening. Was at the hospital at 6:30 AM. At 8:00 AM a procedure for a Radiologist to do wire insertion around breast area. The wires (3 or 4) point to exactly where the tumor is. That was painless because they numb the area. At 10:00 AM second procedure was done under a scanner to find exactly where the sentinel lymph node was so during the surgery they could remove it for a biopsy. 12-noon - time for the lumpectomy - scared."

A short time later, Guy, Janet, Amanda, Vickie and Clint arrived to lend support in any way they could. It was a wonderful experience to have the family with us so they could be with their mom. Being there with Florence and giving her, each in their own little way, loving words of hope, was absolutely wonderful. When the O.R. nurse arrived to take Florence, she could not help but feel the love for Florence emanating from everyone. She asked if she could say a prayer for Florence. She gathered all of us around Florence, and we held hands as she led us in a beautiful prayer. This wonderful experience was very meaningful to all of us, mainly to Florence, giving her hope and confidence. Are there angels around us? Yes, indeed there are!

In Florence's Own Words

"I'll never forget that morning. Janet, Guy Anthony, Clint, Vickie and Amanda were there. And, of course my wonderful, wonderful husband. It was such a secure feeling that I got just knowing they were there. They came in to the little room where I was getting prepped for surgery. Amanda took my hand and said, "How are you doing grandma?" I said "I'm doing fine, especially with all of you here". One of the nurses came in to get me and she asked if we would like her to say a prayer for me. Of course we all said yes. We all held hands while she said a prayer. I was so excited about that, I don't ever remember being in the hospital when a nurse asked if we'd like a prayer said. She had no idea how much that meant to me. I felt safe, again. The family left the room and went to the waiting room.

I remember being rolled down the hallway and seeing them through the window, so I gave them a high-five, and was on my way - Oh my God, I thought . . . I feel so sorry for them."

It was now time to take Florence to surgery. The family wished her well as the nurse wheeled her slowly from her cubicle to the operating room. I walked alongside her with little or no conversation. I just reached out and held her hand. My last glimpse of Florence, as she was wheeled away for surgery, brought tears to my eyes. It is difficult to put into words the helplessness I felt as she was taken through the large double doors with the doors closing behind her. It was a difficult moment for me.

In Florence's Own Words

"It lasted a lot longer (about three and a half hours - was only supposed to be about two hours) than expected because Dr. Wiese went much further than anticipated. He took a lot more out to be on the safe side. It was worth it because the final results after all the surgery was, there was no cancer remaining. I will get final results of all the tests of the tumor they took out on August 21st. Hopefully it will still show no cancer. Can't wait to get those results - scared!!! Guy and the kids were really getting nervous waiting for me to come out of surgery because it wasn't supposed to be that long. Part of the time it took was Dr. Wiese waited for some immediate results from the pathologist who was there to see if he needed to go further, and of course he did."

The next few hours were filled with emotions, anxieties, and uncertainties. Had the cancer spread into her lymph nodes and maybe even to other parts of her body? Would the doctor opt to switch from a lumpectomy to completely removing her breast? Would there be other complications? It was even difficult for me to be near the kids who were sitting patiently in the waiting room; even though they were so supportive with their calming words, "Everything is going to be all right, dad." It was still challenging. I paced up and down the hallway every now and then glancing toward the double doors of the operating room, praying that she would be all right. From time to time, my grandchild Amanda would join me in the hallway and hold my hand as we walked together. She would say, "Grandma is going to be okay, and she will be coming out soon, grandpa." The innocence and love coming from this child have always amazed me. She never ceases to put a smile on my face. I am so proud of her and the rest of our grandchildren. Florence and I are indeed blessed to have them in our lives.

Approximately two hours later, the O.R. nurse came out of the operating room. She told me that Florence was doing fine and that the tumor had been removed. Dr. Wiese was waiting for the pathologist report on the margins before he could close the wound. She said the doctor would speak to me after he was through with the surgery.

I had read enough about the word "margins" to understand what she meant. The pathologist will tell Dr. Wiese how close the tumor is to the margin. The goal is to have clear margins, which means the entire tumor is removed, and no cancer remains. If the margins are not clear, or are too close to the tumor for the surgeon's comfort, the surgeon will go back and remove additional tissue. In Florence's case, the surgeon did indeed go back to remove more tissue, not because it was cancerous but just to make sure all of the cancer had been removed.

Again I waited, walking the hallway, sitting in the waiting room with the family, engaging in small talk about everything and about nothing. It seemed so long since I walked with her when they wheeled her into the O.R. I decided to go downstairs to the hospital chapel. I didn't say anything to the kids about where I was going. They knew I often walked the hallway by myself, so it wasn't a concern to them. I found myself alone in the chapel thinking again about Florence. Would they find cancer in her lymph nodes or other parts of her body? Would she have drains hanging from her arm? Would she have to come back and do this all over again? I thought, "Why Florence? She doesn't deserve this. What could have caused this to happen?" I blurted out loud, "STOP." Embarrassed I looked around the room; it was still empty. No one had heard me. I thought to myself "This is not the time to be negative." I needed PMA! PMA, or positive mental attitude! PMA was what my high school football coach, Armand "Stitch" Vari, said in his numerous emails to Florence after he had learned about her diagnosis. Besides, I wouldn't know anything until I talked with Dr. Wiese. I sat realizing that I was in the hospital chapel, and what I really needed to do was pray. I was learning that talking to God was getting easier. Asking Him to continue to bless and protect Florence, especially now, did bring tears, but it also comforted me. Someone once said, "God promises a safe landing, not a calm passage." I remembered those words then, and I remember them now!

I ran back upstairs to the waiting room and asked the kids if they had heard anything. In the waiting room, there was a telephone used by the physicians to contact family members and to give them the news of there loved ones. The phone had not rung for us in the last three hours. The kids sensed I was getting worried and gave me calming and optimistic words of encouragement. I again walked out to the hallway. This time, however, I saw Dr. Wiese coming through the large double doors of the O.R. We met halfway and he invited my family and me to an auxiliary room next to the waiting room to give us an update. We sat down waiting anxiously to hear what he had to say. The kids stood beside me, giving me the support I really needed.

I introduced Dr. Wiese to the family and immediately asked him, "How's my wife, doctor?" He answered, "Guy, she did very well." He went on to say that her lymph nodes were clear and that he was very optimistic of having removed all of the cancer from her breast. The operation took a little longer because he went back in to remove extra tissue to make sure he had gotten all of the cancer. I was extremely nervous and asked Dr. Wiese about drains. He said that drains weren't necessary because any fluid build-ups would dissolve naturally over time. What great news, I thought to myself, while holding back tears. I looked at my sons, their wives, and Amanda. Each had smiles on his or her face as they stared at me. No words were spoken. Words were not necessary. We knew that God had indeed answered all of the prayers said, by not only the family, but from friends all over the country. This was indeed good news! Florence was cancer-free. I was flooded with relief. But there was also a voice of doubt that said, "Well, maybe it will grow back later; you never are sure..." My faith immediately squashed the doubts because today my faith had worked.

The kids and I hugged each other as they left the hospital knowing that it would be some time before Florence could be released. I waited by the O.R. doors for Florence to be wheeled out, not knowing how she would look or feel. I didn't have long to wait. The large double doors opened, and two nurses navigated her bed with IV's connected to her through the doors. She looked pale; her eyes were closed, but yet there was something beautiful about the way she looked. I wanted so very much to tell her the good news, but this was obviously not the time. I would have to wait until the anesthesia wore off. I followed as they took her to the recovery room, and I waited there as the drugs gradually wore off. The medications that she had been given could remain in her body for up to twenty-four hours. She would not be completely recovered until the anesthetic had been totally eliminated from her body. However, I was still hopeful that I would be able to give her the news about her surgery.

It didn't take long for her to open her eyes and look at me. She was just starting to feel some of the pain and nausea associated with the surgery. I held her hand and called out her name. She stared at me, still very groggy and asked, "How did it go?" With a tear in my eye, choked up a little, I responded. "It went better than expected. It went extremely well. They removed all of the cancer, and the cancer did not spread into your lymph nodes." "Oh, wow really?" she replied, and then she slowly closed her eyes. I was very emotional at that point, and I had to walk out of the room and compose myself. I would learn later that she did not remember our conversation that afternoon.

How Sweet the Sound
Florence you are Cancer Free

CANCER FREE! Those are the two words we have been waiting to hear. I'm sorry to repeat myself, but I have to say it again. "CANCER FREE!"

After visiting the oncologist and the surgeon and listening to them say - "Florence, you are cancer free," it literally knocked me off my chair. You can imagine how Florence was feeling. That, indeed, was a good day.

A little more detail is needed here. As the oncologist was reading the results, and it was indeed lengthy, it occurred to me that the oncologist was slowly telling us that Florence's cancer had been removed. Florence's eyes were getting larger and larger as she was listening to the doctor. In the middle of the report, Florence interrupted the doctor and said - "Are you telling me that the cancer is gone?" The doctor responded, "Florence, you are cancer free." Well, you can imagine the emotions that flooded through Florence at that time. Not me, I kept my emotions in check – yeah, right!

What is astonishing to me is that with the kind of cancer that she was diagnosed with, aggressive stage 2, HER2-positive; the result had been questionable at best. Even the doctor had said, "With this type of cancer, today's results are the best we could have ever asked for! Florence, you did well."

This very exciting news was relayed by email to all of our family and friends. Not only did I give them the above account from the doctor's office, I added the following:

"My dear friends,

I know God has given Florence's doctors a tremendous skill. Florence continues to receive good news after the original diagnosis of Breast Cancer. Over a seven-week period, Florence took all the necessary tests prescribed, and the results were better than anyone expected.

I had always believed Florence needed one extra element in her treatment - prayers! All of you provided that component making all of you a part in Florence's positive outcome. Again, thank you, thank you, and most of all - God Bless all of you."

Florence has always had a unique and inspiring spirit about her, but it took this traumatic experience for me to recognize it. I have no problem acknowledging this spirit, her courage, her perseverance, and her sheer determination to move forward in this long and difficult journey. She has taken the first steps in this quest by removing the cancerous tumor from her body. I am blessed to have her, and I am so very proud of her.

Someone once told me that it takes three things to beat breast cancer. First is the best possible medical treatment. Second is the best possible medical treatment. And third is a positive mental attitude (PMA). If we look at it in the perspective of relative importance, PMA is not burying your head in the sand and saying, "I'm going to get well." It is doing everything within your power to add the best medical treatment possible and to have faith that God is indeed a factor in your care. Without all three, you don't have a chance. But I never thought that the three were enough. I believed, emphatically; you needed one more element - Prayer. So, Florence and I have added, in every instance, prayer to Florence's treatment.

In Florence's Own Words

"Went to see Dr. Shroff for results from surgery. She was explaining everything to us and I had to stop her in the middle and ask if she was telling me I was cancer free. She said yes. Guy and I looked at each other and we both started crying. We couldn't believe what we were hearing. She said she thought I had already seen Dr. Wiese and that he had already told us. Our appointment with Dr. Wiese was right after hers. This was one incredibly happy day for us. When we went to see Dr. Wiese it was great and he made us feel very good. Thank you God!!!"

"How Are You? How's Florence?"

"How are you, how's Florence?" A harmless greeting, but one I deal with all the time. Those friend, and even family members want to know that everything is okay. They want to hear a positive response that everything is fine. How you respond sends all kinds of emotional meanings to them. "I feel great, and Florence is doing well. Thank you for asking." That is my way of not wanting to talk about what Florence may be going through at that moment in time. However, I am respectful of their concern; I just don't have any new news, other than she is doing fine. Sometimes I hesitate mentioning or sharing Florence's cancer experience for fear of how other people might react. I realize everyone reacts differently to difficult or upsetting news so I try to pick the right time in a stress-free environment. "Timing is everything," they say. There have been times where family members and/or friends have difficulty talking about particular topics like cancer, so they try to avoid the conversation. It may be because it is a reminder of a fear they have about cancer or, it triggers a memory of losing a loved one. In most cases, people have been supportive, and I have been appreciative and respectful to their best intentions, but I don't want them to feel sorry for us. On the other hand, I have found unexpected support and encouragement from people that resulted in a much stronger relationship.

What I'm trying to say is, I don't want Florence to be a symbol of a woman that has been going through breast cancer and survived. Although, courageous and inspiring in her battle, she still has always maintained those wonderful attributes of being Florence, - wife, mother, grandmother, a beautiful lady. She was never a cancer victim! She is a cancer survivor and belongs to a club of people who have been touched by cancer in some way. Each of them has their own story, no different than Florence's. There is nothing more inspiring to me than reading about how they survived and dealt with their own unique situations. The stories about their experiences always reminds me of Florence's amazing strength and grace during her journey. And, despite the hardships she endured, she never lost her appreciation for the kindness in this world.

Chemotherapy

On September 12,Th Florence and I met with her medical oncologist, Dr. Shroff, to discuss the chemotherapy protocol Florence will need to undergo. Dr. Shroff generally sees breast cancer patients after the diagnosis, and again after any necessary surgery that follows. As mentioned before, Dr. Shroff specializes in the diagnosis and treatment of cancer. She commonly uses systemic therapy; that is, whole body treatment.

There are a number of ways to treat breast cancer. One is called Systemic Therapy and another is called Local Therapy. Systemic Therapy is the use of drugs that travel in the bloodstream to affect or treat cancer cells. It can be used in combination with Local Therapy. Hormonal treatment, chemotherapy, and targeted therapy are types of systemic therapy. Herceptin is a targeted therapy and will be used as part of Florence's treatment.

Local treatment is directed only at the cancer cells in the breast area. Surgery and radiation are two types of local therapies used for treating breast cancer. When Florence completes her chemotherapy treatments she will start her radiation treatments; and then after she will start hormonal treatments.

Systemic Chemotherapy acts throughout the body in the prevention of the recurrence of the disease as well as in long-term care. It is the use of special drugs that will have a particular destructive effect on Florence's cancer cells.

Why would Florence have to take chemotherapy when she was told she was "cancer free?" Cancer free means the tests she had previously taken, and her recent surgery to remove her cancerous tumor, indicated that she was cancer free. The tests, however, can only see macro cells, not cancer that remains in very small amounts, microscopic metastases cells. Categorizing the extent of the shrinkage of the cancer, Doctors use the term "remission." So, "cancer free" may not be the appropriate statement. Doctors use "complete remission" to categorize a cancer that is no longer evidenced in tests, scans, and x-rays. Cancer free sounds better but "complete remission" is the proper terminology in Florence's case at this point.

Living With Uncertainty

The doctor says you have no signs of cancer now, but can you be sure? Can the doctor be sure? The five "Big" questions are: Will it come back? What are the chances it will come back? How will I know if it has come back? What will I do if it comes back? AND, when will it come back? Florence is now a cancer survivor. She has put the experience behind her. But there is that anxiety the cancer may come back and she will be reliving it all over again.

The recurrence issue is based on the cancer type. When Florence's tissue was removed during the biopsy the pathologist determined if the cancer was indeed present and whether it was in-situ. In-situ is a term used for an early stage of cancer when it is confined to the layer of cells where it began.

The pathologist also assigned a grade to Florence's cancer that was based on how closely the biopsy sample resembles normal breast tissue. The grade helps predict Florence's prognosis. [11]In general, a lower grade number indicates a slower-growing cancer that is less likely to spread, while a higher number indicates a faster-growing cancer that is more likely to spread. Florence's pathologist report indicated ductal carcinoma in-situ, high grade. The patterns of cell growth are rated on a scale from 1 to 3. It is sometimes also referred to as low, medium, and high instead of 1, 2 or 3. A well-organized growth with few cells reproducing is considered grade 1. Disorganized, irregular growth patterns in which many cells are in the process of making new cells is called grade 3. The lower the grade, the more favorable the expected outcome becomes for recovery. [12]At the same time, the higher the grade, the more vulnerable the cancer is to treatments such as chemotherapy and radiation. Therefore, women with a "high" or "grade 3" breast cancer can also feel hopeful about treatment.

How does all of this affect Florence? Even after Florence's initial treatment for early breast cancer, it's possible that her cancer can come back. The term recurrence is used to describe the return of cancer following her surgery either at the same site as the original tumor or somewhere else in her body. If Florence does not receive additional treatment, treatment without chemo or radiation, her risk for a cancer recurrence is highest in the first five years following her diagnosis. As the years go by her risk of a recurrence will drop each year during the next 10 years.

Will Florence's cancer come back at a later date? As described above, there is the possibility the cancer could come back. The good news was the cancer was localized and removed. There was no evidence of metastatic carcinoma, her lymph nodes were clear and the result of the previous scans and the pathology reports also were negative. This could indicate that she was in complete remission. But this was a very aggressive cancer, one that would be very difficult to treat if it returned. Florence, wisely, chose to give up one year of her life to take all of the necessary treatments in order to beat this insidious beast. A decision that will reduce the chances the cancer would return. It was a decision that still overwhelms me. Being diagnosed with cancer, surgery, making decisions on what type of chemo protocol should be used, and now having to deal with the possibility of a recurrence was indeed a very stressful time in her life. But we both felt much better once we knew what we were dealing with, and we finally felt we were taking the right steps in getting rid of this problem.

Cancer Staging

Cancer staging is different from the grade of the cancer and many times it's confusing as to which is which. [13]Stage refers to how far the tumor has invaded into its tissue of origin or progressed beyond it. [14]The stage describes the extent of the cancer in the body. It is based on whether the cancer is invasive or non-invasive, the size of the tumor, how many lymph nodes are involved, and whether it has spread to other parts of the body. [14]The stage of a cancer is one of the most significant factors in determining prognosis and treatment options. Staging of the cancer is based on three main factors. The original tumor size, whether or not the tumor has grown into other nearby areas, and/or whether it has spread to the nearby lymph nodes and to other parts of the body.

Stage 0 - This stage is used to describe non-invasive breast cancer. There is no evidence of cancer cells breaking out of the part of the breast in which it started, or of getting through to or invading neighboring normal tissue. DCIS (Ductal Carcinoma in Situ) is an example of stage 0 cancer.

Stage I – [15]This stage are cancer cells that are breaking through or invading neighboring normal tissue in which the tumor measures up to two centimeters and no lymph nodes are involved.

Stage II – [15]This stage describes invasive breast cancer in which the tumor measures at least two centimeters, but not more than five centimeters, or the cancer has spread to the lymph nodes under the arm on the same side as the breast cancer.

Stage III is divided into sub-categories [16]known as IIIA and IIIB.

Stage IIIA describes invasive breast cancer in which the tumor measures larger than five centimeters, or there is significant involvement of lymph nodes.

Stage IIIB – [16]This stage describes invasive breast cancer in which a tumor of any size has spread to the breast skin, chest wall, or internal mammary lymph nodes. It also includes inflammatory breast cancer, a very uncommon but very serious, aggressive type of breast cancer.

Stage IV – [17]This stage includes invasive breast cancer in which a tumor has spread beyond the breast, underarm, and internal mammary lymph nodes, and a tumor may have spread to the supraclavicular lymph nodes. [18]These are nodes located at the base of the neck, above the collarbone, lungs, liver, bone, or brain.

"Metastatic at presentation" means that the breast cancer has spread beyond the breast and nearby lymph nodes, even though this is the first diagnosis of breast cancer. [18]The was not found when it was only inside the breast. Metastatic cancer is considered stage IV.

Florence's tumor type is called, "Invasive ductal adenocarcinoma and ductal carcinoma in-situ." The situ component represents forty percent of the tumor mass while the adenocarcinoma represents sixty percent of the tumor mass. The size of her tumor was 2.7 x 2.5 x 1.3 cm.

Adenocarcinoma is a type of carcinoma that starts in glandular tissue. These are the tissues that make and secrete a substance. [19]The ducts and lobules of the breast are glandular tissue; they make breast milk, so cancers starting in these areas are sometimes called adenocarcinomas.

Ductal carcinoma in-situ or DCIS, also known as intraductal carcinoma, is the most common type of non-invasive breast cancer. DCIS means that the cancer cells are inside the ducts but have not spread through the walls of the ducts into the surrounding breast tissue.

[19]An invasive cancer is one that has already invaded beyond the layer of cells where it started, as opposed to ductal carcinoma in-situ. Most breast cancers are invasive carcinomas and are the most common type of breast cancer. [20]They start in a milk passage (duct) of the breast, break through the wall of the duct, and invade the fatty tissue of the breast. At this point, they may have the ability to spread, metastasize, to other parts of the body through the lymphatic system and bloodstream. About eight out of ten invasive breast cancers are infiltrating ductal carcinomas. [21]It is not unusual for a single breast tumor to be a combination of these types and to have a mixture of invasive and in-situ cancer. Florence's tumor developed from a ductal carcinoma in-situ to an invasive ductal adenocarcinoma.

Oncotype DX Test

I was talking to my brother-in-law, Tom, who lives in Houston, Texas, updating him on Florence's condition. I discussed with him my concerns regarding the possibility of a recurrence based on her tumor diagnosis. He told me about a recent article he had read about a cancer recurrence test called Oncotype DX that might be of interest to me. [22]The U.S. Food and Drug Administration (FDA) approved the Oncotype DX test in January 2004 for use in patients with node-negative, estrogen-receptor (ER) positive breast cancer.

Oncotype DX is an [22]example of "individualized oncology," whose goals is to match cancer patients with appropriate therapy in order to spare certain patients from the side effects of chemotherapy, improve their quality of life, and provide better outcomes. [22]Based on which of the genes in the breast cancer cells are active, a patient is categorized as having a certain likelihood of recurrence of breast cancer at a distant site by ten years after surgery. In the Oncotype DX test, the categories of risk of recurrence are low, intermediate, and high. By predicting the degree of risk of recurrence, the Oncotype DX test would help Florence and Dr. Shroff select the most appropriate types of post-surgical treatment for her.

However, nothing comes easy when your fighting cancer. As it turns out, my friend, Dr. Bob Baratta, pointed out a discrepancy with the FISH test results and the initial core biopsy. The FISH test indicated the ER was positive and the core biopsy indicated it was negative. I immediately contacted Dr. Shroff to tell her of my findings and my interest in the Oncotype DX test. I told her I had read the surgical pathology report indicating the tumor cells to be approximately fifteen percent positive for ER. However her core biopsy taken on July 10th indicated her ER to be negative. The reason for my concern was if we were to use the Oncotype DX to test for recurrence, her ER would need to be positive for Florence to be a candidate. Secondly, and of most importance to me, why was there a discrepancy? The discrepancy occurred between the sample analyzed from the original biopsy and the sample analyzed from the tumor removed during Florence's surgery. The biopsy sample is less sensitive than the tumor that was removed and, therefore, the pathologist report of ER positive is more accurate. As a result of understanding the results of both pathology reports, Dr. Shroff and I agreed to order the Oncotype DX test.

Dr. Shroff ordered the test and sent the tumor sample to Genomic Health, Inc. in San Francisco.

Genomic Health gives cancer patients and their healthcare providers insights needed to help make quality treatment decisions. The test is designed to help patients, caregivers, and healthcare professionals understand how individualized genomic profiling of tumor tissue may help improve cancer management. The test, developed by Genomic Health, may assist treatment planning by quantifying the likelihood of distant breast cancer recurrence.

The results are taken from a clinical validation study with prospectively defined endpoints involving 668 patients. The patients enrolled in the study were female, stage I, or II, node negative, ER-positive, and treated with tamoxifen. The recurrence score is from 0 to 100.

Florence's recurrence score was seventy-seven. Patients with a recurrence score of greater than fifty in the clinical validation study had an average rate of distant recurrence at ten years of thirty-four percent, the low end being twenty-four percent and the high being forty-four percent, thus an average of thirty-four percent. This is considered a high risk of recurrence. If the score were twenty-five the average rate of recurrence would be approximately twenty-five percent, an intermediate risk. If the score is ten the average rate of recurrence would be approximately seven percent, a low risk. Again Florence's score was seventy-seven with a distant recurrence rate at ten years of approximately thirty-four percent.

Why Chemotherapy?

Earlier I had described terminologies used by doctors like "free of cancer" or "complete remission." Remission is a word doctors often use when talking about cancer. It means there is no sign of the cancer or she is "cancer free." Doctors may be reluctant to say a cancer is 'cured' because some cancers can come back years later. However, the more time that goes by, the less likely it is that a cancer will return. Still, there is always a small chance. In Florence's case, she was told she was cancer free or in complete remission. Complete remission means that the cancer can't be detected on scans, X-rays, or blood tests etc.

OK, we know Florence will always be at risk for a recurrence, and that sometimes she may even be overwhelmed by the fear that it may return. Even so, we're not going to let it in any way interfere with our lives. We know if Florence follows the cancer guidelines she will lessen the chance of a recurrence.

Florence's chemotherapy is being administered with her knowing that there's no evidence of the cancer spreading. This form of treatment is called adjuvant therapy. Adjuvant treatment is given after the primary treatment of removing the tumor to increase the chances of a cure. In Florence's case, adjuvant therapy will include chemotherapy and radiation. It is extra treatment to keep the cancer from returning. Even in the early stages of the disease, microscopic cancer cells can break away from the primary breast tumor and spread through the bloodstream. These cells don't cause symptoms, they don't show up on imaging tests, and they can't be felt during a physical exam. But if they are allowed to spread, they can establish new tumors in other places in the body. Some types of cancer are very sensitive to chemotherapy, but unfortunately others are not. In a cancer that is sensitive to chemotherapy, doctors will use this type of treatment because the chemo drugs will circulate in the bloodstream throughout the body so that it can treat the cancer cells found anywhere in the body. It is what is referred to as 'systemic' treatment. Surgery and radiotherapy are known as 'local' treatments as they only affect the area of the operation or the area the radiotherapy is directed to target.

It is the return of the same type of cancer after Florence's initial treatment that scares us. Therapy for early-stage breast cancer aims to reduce the chance that cancer will return or recur. It is valuable for us to know what the odds are that Florence's cancer may return. That information will help us and her doctors determine whether additional treatment beyond surgery is appropriate.

Breast cancer can recur at any time, but most recurrences occur in the first three to five years after initial treatment. Breast cancer can come back as a local recurrence in the original area or it may be a distant recurrence somewhere else in the body. Signs of local recurrence of breast cancer usually become apparent during mammograms, physical examinations, or self-examinations.

In distance recurrence, the cancer metastasizes or spreads to parts of the body other than the original location. Symptoms such as bone pain, weight loss, and shortness of breath may be signs of distant recurrence. If cancer does metastasize, it commonly spreads to the lungs, bones, liver, or brain. Florence will need to be very diligent, keeping up with all of the precautions her health providers will prescribe for her.

Florence has used every drop of her energy to concentrate on getting rid of her insidious cancer. Many cancers are successfully treated, but generally you have only one chance. If you miss that first chance, if you don't do everything in your power the first time, often there will be no second chance. This is why Florence never looked back, never lost any time questioning why cancer happened to her, and never said, "I wish I would have." What she did say was, "I don't want this thing to ever come back. I want to watch my grandchildren grow and mature, and never have to worry about a recurrence. I'm ready for this journey. I'm ready for chemotherapy, and I intend to stay positive. If the cancer should return, I'll beat it again."

Even after successful surgery, Florence continues her journey down a new road that will be filled with uncertainties. The uncertainties of chemotherapy, and its side effects! We will be together at this juncture of Florence's journey with humor, spirit, hope, and positive thinking. Our good friend Robert Urich once said, "Attitude is everything. It motivates action, which increases productivity and improves morale, which perpetuates a positive attitude." This good man understood what being positive meant. His career, his battle with cancer, his contribution to cancer research, speaks volumes about the character of this man.

Florence Treatment Protocol

Dr. Shroff suggested a chemotherapy treatment that will include Taxotere, Carboplatin, and Herceptin. Florence's chemotherapy recipe is known as TCH. Each letter represents the beginning letter of each of the drugs used. They will be given to Florence in cycles, with each period of treatment followed by a rest period. The chemotherapy will begin on the first day of each cycle, and then there will be time to recover from the effects of the chemotherapy. The period between the therapies is three weeks. The treatment cycles will be over eighteen weeks. Herceptin treatment is once every week and will continue until October, a total of twelve months. After the eighteen weeks of chemotherapy, she will start radiation treatments every day for six weeks.

The above drugs are potent chemotherapy drugs used in cancer treatment and will be the drugs of choice for Florence's treatment. I tried to find out what the side effects would be when she started her chemo treatments, but it was difficult to get a good answer. Everyone is different. No one person has the same symptoms. We would have to wait and see what happens. We do know that Chemotherapy drugs work by attacking cells that are [23]dividing quickly which is why they work against cancer cells. But other cells in the body, such as those in the bone marrow, in the lining of the mouth and intestines, and in hair follicles, also divide quickly. [23]These cells are also likely to be affected by chemotherapy, which can lead to side effects with which Florence will surely have to deal. Fatigue will also be a problem for Florence. It may continue even after her treatments. But, with an exercise program and a plan of conserving her energy, she will overcome this issue.

Taxotere is an anti-cancer chemotherapy drug. Taxotere is classified as a "plant alkaloid approved in the treatment of breast cancer." The amount of Taxotere that Florence will receive will depend on her height and weight, her general health, and the type of cancer being treated.

Taxotere side effects are often predictable in terms of their onset and duration, and the good news is that Taxotere side effects are almost always reversible and will go away after treatment is completed. As she takes Taxotere, there will be an increased risk for infection because her white blood cell count will be low. Also, her red blood cell count will be low which may cause anemia.

[24]Carboplatin belongs to the group of medicines known as alkylating agents. It is used to treat cancer of the ovaries. It may also be used to treat other kinds of cancer, such as breast cancer.

Carboplatin will be administered with the Taxotere. Since it will be combined with the Taxotere, it will be important that Florence receives each one at the proper time. This medicine usually causes nausea and vomiting that sometimes may be severe. However, it is very important that Florence continues to receive the doses, even if she begins to feel ill.

The dose of Carboplatin is different for different patients. Like Taxotere, the dose will depend on a number of things, including Florence's type of cancer and her weight.

Carboplatin will temporarily lower the number of white blood cells in Florence's blood, increasing her chance of getting an infection. It can also lower the number of platelets, which are necessary for proper blood clotting. If this occurs, there are certain precautions Florence can take, especially when her blood count is low.

[25]Carboplatin interferes with the growth of cancer cells, which eventually are destroyed. Since the growths of normal body cells are affected, other side effects will probably occur.

Florence's cancer, as is true in all cancerous tumors, is characterized by cell division, which is not controlled as it is in normal tissue. Normal cells stop dividing when they come into contact with like cells, a mechanism known as contact inhibition. Cancerous cells lose this ability. Cancer cells no longer have the normal checks and balances in place that control and limit cell division. The process of cell division, whether normal or cancerous, is through the cell cycle. The cell cycle goes from the resting phase, through the active growing phases, and then to division.

[25]The ability of chemotherapy to kill cancer cells depends on its ability to halt cell division. Usually, the drugs work by damaging the RNA or DNA that tells the cell how to copy itself in division. If the cells are unable to divide, they die. The faster the cells are dividing, the more likely it is that chemotherapy will kill the cells, causing the tumor to shrink.

Chemotherapy drugs that affect cells only when they are dividing are called cell cycle specific. Chemotherapy drugs that affect cells when they are at rest are called cell-cycle non-specific. The scheduling of chemotherapy is based on the type of cells, the rate at which they divide, and the time at which a given drug is likely to be effective. This is why Florence's chemotherapy is given in cycles.

As we mentioned before, [26]chemotherapy is most effective at killing cells that are rapidly dividing. Unfortunately, chemotherapy does not know the difference between the cancerous cells and the normal cells. The "normal" cells will grow back and be healthy, but in the meantime, side effects will occur. Again, the "normal" cells most commonly affected by [25]chemotherapy are blood cells, the cells in the mouth, stomach and bowel, and the hair follicles, resulting in low blood counts, mouth sores, nausea, diarrhea, and/or hair loss.

Earlier I said Herceptin was not considered a chemotherapy or hormonal therapy drug. It is a type of targeted cancer therapy known as targeted biologic therapy. There are some side effects while taking Herceptin. [26]It can cause flu-like symptoms in about forty-percent of the women who take it. These symptoms may include fever, chills, muscle aches, or nausea. The side effects generally become less severe after the first treatment. Other side effects, including low white or red blood cell counts, diarrhea, and infections, are seen in some women receiving Herceptin in combination with chemotherapy, but are rarely seen in women taking Herceptin alone.

Less common but certainly of concern, is that [26]Herceptin can damage the heart's ability to pump blood effectively. Rarely, in only about 5% of the cases, the heart damage is bad enough that women can experience stroke or life threatening congestive heart failure. This is a condition whereby the heart can't pump blood effectively.

Before Florence started her Herceptin treatment, Dr. Shroff checked any health conditions that could increase her chances of having serious heart problems. Florence reviewed her health history with Dr. Shroff and there was no indication of any history of heart problems. However, Dr. Shroff ordered a MUGA scan, which takes a moving picture of her heart pumping blood following an injection of a radioactive substance. Even though heart failure is less likely to occur the longer Florence takes Herceptin, Dr. Shroff will still order heart-monitoring tests every six months or so. Also, during the Herceptin treatment, Florence will continually be monitored for any decreasing heart function, even though the severe side effects are relatively rare.

Florence will continue to be monitored. Her health care professionals will check her regularly while she is taking these chemicals. They will monitor the side effects and check her response to the therapy. Dr. Shroff will also order periodic blood work to monitor her complete blood count (CBC), as well as the function of her other organs, such as her kidneys and liver.

Alternative Treatments

Florence has been told horror stories by well-meaning friends about someone they knew who had taken chemotherapy. Some even suggested she not take any chemo; it would not be worth it, as she would suffer horribly from the treatments. Florence and I would shrug off these stories believing her team of doctors could combat most of the side effects. Besides, in the last ten years, there have been great strides giving patients better outcomes.

Florence will take one treatment at a time, knowing well it won't be pleasant, but she also knows there is an end-time and all of this will pass. Still, it bothered me that people would believe the chemotherapy was deadly, and would not help. Some even suggested taking a holistic approach to Florence's cancer treatment. "Holistic or alternative treatment, what is that all about?"

I was introduced to the world of complementary and alternative medicine, known as CAM, by a friend whose wife had been diagnosed with breast cancer in January. The news came to me by email seven months after her diagnosis and about two weeks after Florence was diagnosed. The cancer was interductal carcinoma in stage II. This was all I knew about his wife's condition. My immediate response was, "How did her surgery go? What were the follow up treatment?" He answered, "There was no surgery other than her biopsy! The only treatment she was taking was started in Poland by a holistic healer named Momczilo Bozovic. "Holistic?" I responded. "What do you mean, holistic?"

My friend was very distraught and frustrated, specifically at not being able to convince his wife to seek medical attention. He said, "For the last seven months, it has been exasperating, and there have been times she would insist on not talking about it at all." I said to him, "Your wife is in denial." I continued to tell him the feeling of disbelief is sometimes accompanied by a wish to shut out and deny the news and pretend that it is not happening. This is a normal reaction to a very distressing and difficult situation. Florence did not experience the denial syndrome when she was first diagnosed because she felt the thing inside of her didn't belong there and she wanted it removed immediately. She made every effort to move as quickly as possible and plan a treatment program for herself.

I told him his wife's denial could be helpful in dealing with the very threatening and overwhelming news. It could help her to cope with her situation. The danger is, however, the emotions have persisted over the last seven months, and it sounds as if it caused a breakdown in communications between the two of them. I told him, "The cancer is causing the emotional experience she needs to talk to a medical professional. It could be the first step towards dealing with her cancer and moving forward to getting proper treatment as soon as possible. Waiting seven months to get medical treatment after being diagnosed with breast cancer can be very serious, especially if your wife has an aggressive cancer."

The world of alternative treatments is indeed a world unto itself, where healers tout the benefits of all sorts of unconventional therapies for cancer patients.

A 1998 editorial in the [27]Journal of the American Medical Association said:

"There is no alternative medicine. There is only scientifically proven, evidence-based medicine supported by solid data, or unproven medicine, for which scientific evidence is lacking. Whether a therapeutic practice is "Eastern" or "Western," is unconventional or mainstream, or involves mind-body techniques or molecular genetics, is largely irrelevant except for historical purposes and cultural interest. We recognize that there are vastly different types of practitioners and proponents of the various forms of alternative medicine and conventional medicine, and that there are vast differences in the skills, capabilities, and beliefs of individuals within them and the nature of their actual practices. Moreover, the economic and political forces in these fields are large and increasingly complex and have the capability for being highly contentious. Nonetheless, as believers in science and evidence, we must focus on fundamental issues, namely, the patient, the target disease or condition, the proposed or practiced treatment, and the need for convincing data on safety and therapeutic efficacy."

[27]Arnold Relman, M.D. former editor of The New England Journal of Medicine, has expressed similar thoughts:

"There are not two kinds of medicine, one conventional and the other unconventional that can be practiced jointly in a new kind of "integrative medicine." Nor, as Andrew Weil and his friends also would have us believe,

are there two kinds of thinking, or two ways to find out which treatments work and which do not. In the best kind of medical practice, all proposed treatments must be tested objectively. In the end, there will only be treatments that pass that test and those that do not, those that are proven worthwhile and those that are not."

[27]John Farley, Ph.D., professor of physics at the University of Nevada, Las Vegas, commented,

"Integrative" medicine is purportedly combining alternative and mainstream approaches to medicine. The claim is that integrative medicine provides the best of both approaches. This may sound reasonable, but actually it is not. Suppose that the "integrative" approach were to spread beyond medicine, and were to be more broadly adopted by other disciplines in the sciences. The biologists would "integrate" creationism with Darwinian evolution, while the chemists would integrate alchemy into modern scientific chemistry. The geologists would integrate the belief that the world is only 6000 years old (and flat) with modern dating of rocks. Physicists would integrate perpetual motion machines with the conservation of energy and the laws of thermodynamics. And the astronomers would integrate astrology and astronomy. Of course, this is ridiculous. It's not a good idea to integrate nonsense with valid scientific knowledge.

[27]*The "alternative movement" is part of a general societal trend toward rejection of science as a method of determining truths. This movement embraces the post modernist view that science is not necessarily more valid than pseudoscience. In line with this philosophy, "alternative" proponents assert that scientific medicine (which they mislabel as allopathic, conventional, or traditional medicine) is but one of a vast array of health-care options. "Alternative" promoters often gain public sympathy by portraying themselves as a beleaguered minority fighting a self-serving, monolithic "Establishment."*

I may have stepped over the boundaries by inserting a controversial subject, alternative healing and treatments as it applies to breast cancer. I tried to gain knowledge of Florence's cancer, by not only talking to our doctors, but also by reading many articles and research papers. During the research, I found many web sites purporting cancer cures and remedies. I realize the importance to learn what scientific studies have discovered about cancer therapy, but I also learned it was not a good idea to use an alternative therapy simply because of something you have seen on the internet or because others have told you that it worked for them.

I believe there is some rules in science that scientist, engineers, and others adhere to. One rule is who ever makes a claim bears the burden of proving the claim. It is their responsibility to conduct studies and to report their results in detail. It can then be evaluated, and confirmed by others, who are qualified and have the expertise in the field, and who use scientific standards. Instead of conducting scientific studies, many practitioners use anecdotes and testimonials to promote their claims. What really sets alternative medicine apart is that it has not been scientifically tested. [28]Many promoters of alternative medicine believe the scientific method is simply not applicable to their remedies.

In my case, I want to see studies done by prominent institutions, by the best peer-reviewed medical journals, and approvals by the Food and Drug Administration (FDA). I've yet to find herbs or mixtures of herbs, and healing methods such as homeopathy, having any clinical evidence of effectiveness. There is a persistent argument that suggests when using a product, if you feel better it proves the product has worked or is working. Forget that most ailments resolve themselves and those that persist can have variable symptoms. Another drawback of individual success stories is that they don't indicate how many failures might occur for each success. [29]People who are not aware of these facts tend to give undeserved credit to "alternative" methods. Studies have shown that some herbal products interact with drugs and can have a wide range of unintended effects.

Dr. Shroff told Florence and me a story where a patient of hers was being treated with chemotherapy and did not tell her that she was involved in alternative treatments. Her patient was taking a mixture of herbs, which caused a serious interaction with the chemo drugs she was taking. She almost died from the combined treatment.

[30]The Federal Trade Commission (FTC) has a story about a company based in British Columbia making false claims that it can treat cancer by device to kill cancer cells. The Commission has charged CSCT, Inc. that it used its Internet [30]this treatment to consumers in the United States and elsewhere. According to the FTC, the defendants charged consumers $15,000 up front for several weeks of "treatments" with the

electromagnetic device. Consumers must travel at their own expense to Tijuana, Mexico for these treatments. [31]The FTC complaint asserts that the treatments consist of exposing consumers to the "Zoetron" machine, a device that purportedly [30]uses a pulsed magnetic field to heat and kill cancer cells. The FTC alleges that the device cannot kill cancer cells, and that the claims made for this therapy are false. [30]The FTC asserts that on some occasions consumers have foregone more traditional cancer therapies such as chemotherapy or radiation and undertaken the CSCT therapy instead.

Although I am respectful of those who truly believe in alternative treatments, I would suggest to them to try the two methods, Homeopathy and a medical treatment process where hundreds of thousands of scientists share the same observations and beliefs. I would also suggest one not delay seeking advice from a qualified licensed medical professional about treatment for your cancer. [35]Talk to your doctor, pharmacist, or other health provider about any medicines you take, as well as any dietary supplements you're using or thinking about using. Though some doctors have limited knowledge of herbal products and other supplements, they have access to the most current research and can help monitor your condition to ensure that no serious interactions occur.

I cannot overly stress how important the above recommendation is. So, please, please consult your qualified [36]licensed medical professional or appropriate health care provider about the applicability of any opinions or recommendations with respect to your own symptoms or medical conditions. Check out any health claims with a reliable source, such as the National Institutes of Health's Office of Dietary Supplements, a public health or scientific organization like the American Cancer Society and your health provider.

All of the above is an opinion formed by the research I've done. It is not meant to discourage the reader from undertaking conventional treatments for your cancer. I'm hopeful it will support the readers to undertake a smarter and a more effective approach to beat their cancer.

Chemotherapy Starts

From the moment Florence was diagnosed with cancer, chemotherapy was a frightening word. The fear was mostly emotional. You push the poison through your body knowing you might destroy the cancer cells, but it will also destroy the healthy cells. We both had decided to get used to the term, "chemotherapy," the other "C" word. We would repeat the word all the time, and it was amazing how we got used to the word. Still though, it was scary to Florence, and deep down it was scary to me, too!

Chemo drugs are kept in a sealed room, usually stored in a room behind a glass window. Nurses wear a thick, elbow length rubber gloves loading clear plastic bags with the name of the chemical written on the bag. The treatment involves intravenous liquid chemicals delivered directly into the bloodstream. After the treatment you can expect to get nausea, baldness, aching bones, headaches, mental fogginess, blurred vision, and a vulnerability to infection. This is what we know. We know because we've been there. Florence and I, on many occasions, escorted my mother to the cancer treatment center and saw first hand my mom's treatment and the resulting side effects.

I can understand why Florence was scared. She knows it makes patients sick and miserable, yet I know it promises the hope of survival. With all of the negativism toward the chemotherapy, I understand why Florence had a lot of preconceived negative thoughts.

We recognize that the term "chemotherapy" conjures up certain unpleasant images in cancer treatment. But we've learned "chemotherapy" simply means treatment, using drugs, as opposed to treatment by radiation therapy, surgery, gene modification, or other techniques.

The whole process can create a sense of helplessness, but it intensifies our total trust in Florence's Oncologist. It's not going to be easy for her, but I know she can do it.

Paranormal Events

Florence was blessed to receive emails from friends who had unforgettable experiences dealing with cancer in their family. The emails were consistent with support of Florence's decision to go through the chemotherapy treatments. Their experiences provided so much more credibility in their notes to Florence.

Each of us can remember, vividly, the loss of a loved one. So many of us have stories we will never forget during the time our loved one said good-bye. Florence has had, what I believe to be, unique experiences with individuals at the moment or immediately after their individual passing. People call these "Paranormal Events." I'm not sure. I know people have these kinds of mystical moments, but often they are dismissed. These things just don't happen! Hmm! Maybe, if everybody talked about them, how different our attitudes about life and death might be.

Two experiences with individuals and their stories have touched us and left indelible marks in both of our lives. The first was with our sister-in-law, Barbara Jo Hyland.

There are several reasons for including Barbara Jo Hyland in this book. Not only because she was a devoted mother and wife to Florence's brother Jim, but also a wonderful sister-in-law who left an unforgettable imprint in Florence's life. Barbara Jo was another member of our family who bravely fought cancer, finally losing the battle in 1991. Barbara Jo's acceptance of her destiny has been an inspiration to many who deal with this insidious disease every day. One remarkable event I will never forget left Florence with a loving expression of Barbara's generosity the first few minutes after she had passed away. A powerful statement to Florence that she has not left us, but instead, continues to live with us in spirit. This wonderful gift to Florence, given the very moments after her death, has never been forgotten. Florence has said, "When I recall Barbara, I feel those moments then and now." It is a part of Florence's history and has made her stronger facing her own adversities. Barbara Jo's story dealing with metastatic cancer inspires all of us to remember what courage means.

During the afternoon before Barbara died, Florence and I were privileged and honored to be at her bedside with her two sons, and her husband and caretaker, Jim. Even though there was sadness in the expectation that soon Barbara would be leaving us, to describe those moments cannot help, but spark emotions. Her bed was deliberately moved to take advantage of the views through the bedroom window of their waterfront home. Barbara enjoyed very much watching all the aquatic animals and the beautiful sunsets. She often talked about the dolphins playing in the water and the seagulls flying in and around the boats.

The minute Barbara passed; an extraordinary event occurred. A group of dolphins appeared within twenty feet of their boat dock. The dolphins were jumping in and out of the water in circles. This event continued for a few moments and then they disappeared. The family had seen the dolphins months earlier some distance from the home, but never as close as that day, or as many dolphins. Was there a message for us? Maybe! We all have different interpretations of the event, even to this day. Yet, another remarkable event was just about to happen.

After Barbara left us, and the family had said goodbye, an extremely emotional time as you can imagine, Florence was left alone with Barbara. It was difficult for her to leave Barbara by herself, and she needed more time to be with her. Florence would not tell anyone about those moments until a few days later as we were preparing for the funeral.

Florence and I were walking in a parking lot on the way to pick up groceries when Florence stopped and turned staring at me. I asked her, "What's wrong?"

She responded, "I want to share something that happened to me, but you're going to think I'm silly."

I asked, with high expectation, "What, what happened? What's wrong?"

She went on to say, "Remember when I was alone with Barbara after she passed away?"

"Yes," I said, "You were with her for about forty-five minutes."

Florence continued, "I was holding and stroking Barbara's hand saying a prayer or two when a glowing light emerged between her and me. I can't describe it. It was white and soft, almost like a cloud, and it was very bright."

I pressed Florence for more details and started to be analytical with my questions. Florence was at a loss as to what happened and appeared to be distraught about the event.

She continued, "The light was there for only seconds, but I felt a deep sense of warmth as it glowed. It seemed to radiate around us. I then felt as if a hand was touching my shoulder and I swear, I knew it was Barbara. Guy, I was so taken back by the moment. I can't explain it."

"Why didn't you tell me earlier?" I asked?

She said, "I was somewhat embarrassed and thought everyone would think I was silly."

I said to her, "Florence, you should tell this story to Jim as soon as you get a chance. He deserves to hear it. It is an amazing story and he will thank you for it."

Sharing this story with you, the reader, transported me to that week, an emotional one with messages of love and affection pouring in from everywhere. But the story needed to be shared with the family before I could publish it. I needed to know that Florence's brother and nephews would feel that the story of Barbara Jo was accurate and would be meaningful to so many dealing with their cancer. Doing so, I was concerned that I would bring back the memories and emotions of that week. However, I went ahead and sent a draft of this segment of my story to young Jim, Barbara Jo's first born. His reply was extraordinary. He wrote the following,

"I remember the day. I think it was just before noon, my mother was not doing well and taking a turn for the worse. The priest had already come to give the Anointing of the Sick, and the doctor to prescribe higher doses of pain medication. I had spent the night before sleeping on the floor next to her bed, which had been set up in the TV Room. I had just taken a break and was sitting in the kitchen when someone said that things looked bad and that I should come back quickly. As I headed across the Great Room I looked out at the water. It was a particularly beautiful, sunny day. Ironic, I thought. Then I noticed the water was very active. I stopped and it took me a minute before I realized that it was actually a huge number of dolphins breaking the surface, all seeming to swim past the dock from left to right, in the direction of the TV room. It was just coming up to 12-noon, so we all prayed the Angelus together at my mother's bedside, while she struggled with her breathing. I

was not able to speak at the time, but in my heart I was shouting "I Love You!" While others around me began to cry and say goodbye, I held my breath, waiting for the last minute miracle. I felt abandoned by God. I felt He didn't come through for someone who did a lot for Him and His Church. I was angry with God! Only minutes after finishing our prayer she was gone.

When Aunt Florence later told us about the light in the room, I began to cry; first because I wasn't there when it happened, but then out of joy, because I realized that she was witnessing a heavenly promise carried out. She was there, at the hour of death, when in the light of God, with the plentitude of His graces, my mother was received into heaven. God had not abandoned us, but in fact was right there at my mother's side right through to the "bitter end" (even after I had left the room). I was no longer angry. I understood. I couldn't think of anything better than knowing that my mother was not alone, but that she had us, and particularly Aunt Florence with her to accompany her, holding her hand as she approached heaven's door.

Aunt Florence was given something special in that room, that nobody else got. My mother had already accepted her destiny and was ready for what was to come next. We were the ones who needed the time. But I believe that during that time, when everybody else had left the room, the "glow" was passed on. Aunt Florence saw the light of Hope, first hand. She witnessed the power of the Divine. I believe she was given the extra strength at that time, to take-up the cross of cancer where my mother left it, unable to carry it any further. To carry it right through, with the help, support and prayers of all of us, and all of those who passed on before her."

- Jim Hyland III

Barbara Jo and her husband, Jim, were very active in providing religious pilgrimages to a little village in the Catholic parish of Medjugorje. The parish is situated in Herzegovina, fifteen miles southwest of Mostar where today approximately 4000 inhabitants live. [37]Bosnia and Herzegovina make up a triangular-shaped Republic, about half the size of Kentucky, on the Balkan Peninsula. The Bosnian region in the north is mountainous and covered with thick forests. The Herzegovina region in the south is largely rugged, flat farmland. It has a narrow coastline stretching thirteen miles along the Adriatic Sea. The pastoral care of the parish is confided to Fr. Jozo Zovko O.F.M. a priest of the Herzegovinian Franciscan Province of the Assumption of Mary.

Since 1981, in Medjugorje, the Blessed Virgin Mary has been appearing and giving messages to the world. [38]She tells us that God has sent her to this world and in these years she is spending with us, is a time of Grace granted by God. In her own words she tells us, "I have come to tell the world that God exists. He is the fullness of life, and to enjoy this fullness and peace, you must return to God."

When the apparitions started, the lives of witnesses, six visionaries, and the entire parish, including pilgrims from all over the world were changed, and so was Barbara Jo Hyland.

Barbara Jo's extraordinary story is part of the millions of pilgrims of all faiths, from all over the world, who have visited Medjugorje. She organized trips to Medjugorje, bringing countless nonbelievers to be converted and healed.

In the last year of her life she was deeply moved by the kindness and love of so many people. During that year, the last year she would be with us, she wrote a letter to Fr. Jozo in Tihaljina, Yugoslavia. The following is what she said:

"Dear Fr. Jozo,

I am feeling very well physically; I have no pain; I have no feeling of illness. This is amazing considering the rapid pace my cancer is running through my body!! I now also have it in my blood and my lungs and other than sometimes I feel a little out of breath, I feel great!! I have never been so content, so happy, or so peaceful!!

The whole experience has been a real gift for which I am very grateful!! I don't know how to explain to people that I am fine. I am wrapped in the most wonderful warm feeling I have ever experienced and I love every minute of it!! It is like a constant hug from my best friend. I really hope and pray this is the contentment most people feel when they are confronted with their destiny - it is just the most incredible experience of my life!! And, you know that I freely admit that I consider my whole life to have been very exciting, fascinating, wonderful happening - day after day. I still couldn't ask for another thing... I have had far more than any one person deserves – but, I love it. Every morning I wake up to the most beautiful days so far and look forward to living each day to see what will happen next. It is just wonderful!!

Now, if I could convince those around me that there is really nothing to fear and that the 'glow' they see in me is really happy anticipation, they would feel so much better!! There are so many people praying for me, I can feel the power of, the prayer! I am sure the prayer is what is making everything so easy for me!! (God knows He is dealing with a coward!!). As one lady said to me at the Conference, 'You have made us all think a little more seriously about our lives and the importance of our prayer life.' Wasn't that a nice thing to hear!! I love you!! Pray for me!"

- Barbara Jo Hyland

The "glow" Barbara talks about is, maybe, the "glow" Florence experienced the afternoon Barbara Jo passed away.

Florence and Robert Urich

Heather Manzies Urich, wife of actor Robert Urich, was one example of the kindness, love and support given to Florence. Heather played Louisa, one of the Von Trapp children, in the film version of "THE SOUND OF MUSIC." Her messages to Florence on how she dealt with her husband's chemotherapy treatments were helpful and enlightening. Heather is also an ovarian cancer survivor.

I remember when Robert was diagnosed with Synovial Cell Sarcoma, and how he then became an advocate for cancer research. This involvement led to establishing the Robert Urich Fund for Sarcoma Research. Because of this commitment he and Heather helped raise thousands of dollars, and gave hope to thousands of stricken people. Florence and I participated in the fund raising events held at the Sherwood Country Club in Thousand Oaks, California. In 2002, over $500,000 was raised in one weekend for The Robert Urich Fund.

In 1977, Burt Reynolds, often called "Bud" by his close friends, introduced us to Robert Urich at his ranch in Jupiter, Florida. Bud, in those days, funded a community theater in Port Salerno Florida, which later moved to Jupiter, Florida, and became the Burt Reynolds Dinner Theater. Later still, the theatre was renamed the Maltz Jupiter Theater.

Florence and I had the opportunity to work with the theater, donating and producing the playbill for the Reynolds theater productions. The relationship started a friendship with him and some of his actor friends, including Sally Field, James Best and others. Robert Urich and I hit it off immediately as both of us shared a common interest in scuba diving, fishing, and most importantly, family values. When he was performing at the Burt Reynolds Dinner Theater he would find time to dive with me in the waters off Stuart, Florida. Likewise, when Florence and I were in California, we would take dive trips off the Channel Islands National Park. We would often visit with him and his wife at their Canada lakeside home.

Robert was an almost constant presence on television during his career. In fact, according to the trivia book "10,000 Answers: The Ultimate Trivia Encyclopedia," Robert holds the record for starring in the most TV shows, with fifteen. He was awarded the 2059th star on the Hollywood Walk of Fame in December 1995.

January 2002, Bob and I were discussing a novel I had written, titled *ADX*, and the possibility of taking the storyline to television. I felt if anyone could pull it off; he could. On April 15, 2002, I called him to follow up on its status. The person who answered his house phone was the children's nanny who seemed to be very distraught and handed the phone to a friend of his. His friend said that, Bob was in the hospital in critical care, and that he was not expected to recover. He told me that, in August 2001, Bob's cancer had come back, and during the last eight months the cancer had spread to his lungs. I was shocked hearing this news since Bob had never indicated to me he had been diagnosed a third time. In fact, he and I had been fishing together in Canada in the summer of 2001, and he never gave me a hint of his condition. One day we were out on the lake on the way to his favorite fishing hole when I poked him in the shoulder and said, "Bob, you would tell me if you were sick wouldn't you?"

He replied. "Guy, I'm fine and I would tell you." Two months later he would start his third and last battle with this disease.

I told Florence the sad news, and we immediately made preparations to go to California. Then early the next morning, Monday, April 16, Florence awakened me at 4:15 and said to me "Bob died." I was angry at her for making the comment and said, "Why would you wake me at 4:15 AM to tell me that? How would you know?

Florence said, "I had a dream and felt a breath of air on my face and somehow I felt it was Bob's last breath." Skeptical as I am about things like this, I said to her that it was silly to think that and that she was just dreaming. At 6:30 AM, my daughter-in-law called to tell us that there was a "Breaking News Alert." We turned on the local TV station to hear the message, "Robert Urich had died." We were both in shock. The station went on to say, "Robert Urich died in Thousand Oaks, California, surrounded by family and friends, according to Robert's publicist. The actor announced in 1996 that he was suffering from Synovial cell sarcoma, a rare cancer that attacks the body's joints. He underwent several treatments to fight the cancer during the last years of his life."

We simply couldn't believe it. As the day progressed and more news sources were broadcasting his obituary and tributes, we both felt very sad that our friend, a good and decent man, was gone.

The astonishing part of this story is Florence's waking me up at 4:15 AM on the 16th of April to tell me Bob had died.

In Heather's own words

"I was [39]holding Bob in my arms, and I whispered in his ear that he could let go - he could come into my heart, where it was safe, warm, and he would not hurt anymore. It was time for you to go home, I said. I kissed him, and as I did, he took his last breath, into my mouth and there he will live in my heart forever."
- Heather Menzies Urich

Hearing a story that potentially fulfills an issue of human need, - healing and closure, can be brittle and uncomfortable. It reveals the depths of the distress, yet it is a visible and concrete fulfillment of a wonderful relationship, a journey Heather and Robert Urich had taken together.

Robert Urich had taken his last breath and died at 1:15 AM that morning, California time, the exact time Florence had the dream at 4:15 AM, Eastern Standard Time. Was this a paranormal event?

Florence and I spent a week with Heather and the Urich family. His funeral was at St. Charles Borromeo Catholic Church in North Hollywood on April 19, 2002.

Robert was buried in Canada at their waterfront summer cottage. A few days after the burial ceremony, during a spectacular sunset, Emily, Heather's daughter, and Heather, were watching the sunset when a beautiful white Crane landed on their boat dock. They watched with amazement as the Crane slowly walked toward them. Both of them did not know the significance of the Crane at the time, but in some way they knew it was a message. As Emily wrapped her arms around her mother, she said, "Dad is sending us a message Mom." After a few minutes, and as the sun set in the evening sky, the Crane flew away.

Our friendship with Heather and her children continues today. Her friendship has been very rewarding to Florence and me. She often sends emails to us with loving support and optimistic messages.

"C" Day

On October 4th, Florence and I started our day early by enjoying breakfast together. Each of us tried not to talk about what was about to happen. Of course, her breakfast was somewhat limited since today she would begin her first cycle of chemotherapy. It was obvious we were both nervous and didn't know what the treatment itself was going to be like.

It's hard to describe the initial reaction. I wanted so badly to give her a big hug and to congratulate her on her decision to undergo treatments that would last more than a year. But this was not the time, and even if I did, I would have certainly lost it. This was a day, one of many, to be as strong as I could be, to be confident, and to be supportive. No tears! Reign in the emotions.

The drive to the center took twenty minutes. Very little was said on the way. We listened to the news on the car radio, but I'm not sure we were really listening. This was going to be a day the both of us would never forget. I have said this so many times before in this book, but I need to say it again. I am so impressed with Florence for taking on this battle with an attitude that is so inspirational to so many of her friends and family - and to me.

Florence entered the treatment center and signed in at the reception desk. They were expecting her. After a brief consultation with Dr. Shroff as to what she should expect, she walked into the treatment room - and I followed.

This was not the first time Florence had visited a chemotherapy center. As a wonderful caretaker for my mother, Florence would take her to the treatment center; the same center Florence now finds herself in. . . not as a caretaker, but now as a cancer patient. It is incredible to me to know this cancer treatment center was where my mom had visited, taking chemotherapy the last year of her life. Now my wife will be sitting, probably, in the same chair my mom sat in during her battle with cancer. In some ways, knowing my mom was here before, allows us to reflect and to know Florence has a very special angel watching over her.

When we walked from the waiting room and through the doors that led into the treatment room, I was stunned. I can't imagine what Florence was thinking. I really don't know how to describe my first reaction.

There were patients sitting in chairs along a wall, windows behind them. There were expressions of pain; there were tears, and yet some had smiles on their faces. Nurses were running around waiting on and attending to the patients, and the chemo bags hanging on poles. Maybe one of the reasons it hit me hard was because I realized this was going to be a new experience for Florence, a new world she would now be entering.

Escorted over by one of the nurses, Florence sat in a reclining lounge chair, what is referred to as a "chemo chair." There is an IV pole next to her chair on one side where the bags of fluids are hanging. Each bag has a clear tube connected to a tee and from there hangs a single tube connected to her previously installed intravenous access port. Florence sits patiently there while the drugs slowly enter her body through the IV line and to her port. I watch closely, taking notes as to the prescribed dosage of each bag. There are three bags; one for Taxotere one for Carboplatin and one for Herceptin, the chemicals that have been determined to reduce the risk of Florence's having a recurrence. Blood is drawn, and medicine is delivered by placing a needle through the overlying skin into the port or reservoir. I thank the Lord that this part of her treatment is painless.

The previous day, Florence started a steroid treatment program as part of her chemotherapy. Each chemotherapy session starts the day before, the day of chemo, and the day after chemo, with Dexamethasone, the steroid treatment. This drug is unlike the "anabolic" steroids that we hear about regarding sports medicine; these are "catabolic" steroids. Instead of building the body up, they are designed to break down stored resources (fats, sugars and proteins) so that they may be used as fuels in times of stress. Cortisone would be an example of a related hormone with which most people are familiar. We're hopeful the steroid treatment will help prevent Florence from being sick and that it will also help the chemo drugs to work better in eliminating any cancer cells from her body.

I find myself out of place here feeling I might be in someone's way. Maybe the nurses and even the patients are wondering what I'm doing. The room is small, so I find a little space against the wall across from where Florence is seated. I stare at her watching every move worrying if the chemo drugs might cause an unknown reaction, a reaction no one is expecting. I try to make light of the situation, but deep down I feel overwhelmed by everything around me. Then it happens - Florence breaks down. With tears in her eyes, trembling and very emotional she looks at me, whispering, "I'm scared." I quickly move over to her, hold her hand and say, "There's nothing to be scared of honey, all of this will be over soon."

There was utter silence in the room. Other patients knew what she was going through, they had been there and remembered their first chemo treatment. I continued to hold Florence's hand and tried my best to console her. It was indeed another difficult moment for me. I felt a strong urge building up inside me to let loose the floodgates. But these feelings needed to be contained and controlled even though the dam door had opened a little; I wasn't going to allow a meltdown to occur. I repressed my emotions and tried to be as strong as I could as I coped with a tough situation.

Florence composed herself and settled in, realizing she had indeed entered a whole new world. She had crossed the line when she went through the doors of the cancer treatment center. She now belonged in that world, and I was a part of it in my own small way.

I wondered what she was experiencing as the fluids entered her body, drip by drip. She told me she had one sensation, a metallic taste in her mouth. I knew there would be other side effects; some will not be fun, but I knew this brave lady would tolerate all of them.

Florence felt fine during the first few hours after the chemotherapy. Usually, we were told, some reaction occurs about four to six hours later. However, Florence's reaction didn't start until some twenty-four hours later. We both understood that every person experiences chemotherapy differently. There would be both physical and emotional experiences. The side effects for each person from the chemotherapy are different, and different drugs can cause different side effects. We are fortunate that the science of cancer treatment has advanced, and so has managing the treatment of the side effects.

After three and a half hours, Florence had completed her first chemotherapy treatment. She came through the doors from the treatment room with a smile of relief on her face. I looked at her and raised my hand indicating there were only five more treatments to go. She stops and says, "Wow, five more to go. I never looked at it that way." I asked, "How did it go?" She replied, "Guy, it really wasn't as bad as I expected. In fact, it went well. Hopefully, the remaining treatments will be as easy as this one."

The day after each treatment she will get a subcutaneous injection of Neulasta to keep her white blood cells (WBC) count from dropping as a result of the chemo drugs. White blood cells help your body fight off illness and infections. The Neulasta drug will be used to help stimulate her bone marrow to make white blood cells when she is not able to produce them on her own. Florence found these shots to be very painful, and she would continue to have pain in her bones for the next few days following each injection.

This is Florence's world now, one she will get used to. But, I wonder what this experience will be like for her? Each time she walks through those doors, she'll be a stranger in a strange land. What will she see that I won't see? What will she feel that I won't feel? Nevertheless, I'll still be waiting for her when she comes back through those doors.

We now wait for the side effects to show up. Many people have told us horrific stories about chemotherapy and warned us of the side effects. We understood it would be difficult knowing there would be some side effects from the drugs, the poison, as some would say. Florence had made up her mind though, and with the help of prayers, she will continue to move forward with the treatments.

In Florence's Own Words

"TODAY'S THE DAY! I met Dr. David Diamond (radiologist) today at 8:00 AM and that was a real upper. The radiation doesn't sound bad at all. Should not have any side effects and it only takes 15 minutes or so to do. But that's about 5/6 months from now. I felt very good after meeting Dr. Diamond. He's very smart and knew everything about me when he first came in, so he did his homework. He also knew Jan Jablanski and her husband David. They both met him in residency and both helped him through that.

Then we met with Dr. Shroff at 1:00 PM and went through everything that was going to happen today. She made me feel very comfortable and she also is very smart. Thank God Guy is always there, there's a lot to remember. The Herceptin may not have to be every week after the six-chemo treatments (along with Herceptin), it may be every three weeks instead. So that was also good news. As Guy said to me yesterday, "after today I only have five more treatments to go on chemo/Herceptin" and that really hit home. So here I am today with only five treatments left (yea!).

When I actually walked into the treatment room, I got another slap across the top of my head. I just couldn't believe what I was getting ready to do. So I lost it, but only for a few minutes. I actually think those tears helped me, I felt a little relieved. But you take a look at the people in the treatment room, you're in another world, and it is quite scary.

Anyway, I'm doing well so far. It will be interesting how I'll be doing tonight and tomorrow."

Florence's Character!

I'm not sure when it is a good time to talk about my wife's personality and her belief system. I alluded to it a few times already, but maybe this is one of those times I should elaborate.

Making a decision to give up one full year of her life to fight this cancer is not surprising to me. During the past year, she often said, "I want to see my grandchildren grow and mature into young adults. I want to share with them all of the wonderful opportunities they would have, thanks to my sons and their wives. No one can be blessed more than I for God giving me this wonderful family. I will fight this cancer, and I will win." This is the character of my wife, Florence. She has set her priorities - starting with the love of God and her love of family.

Throughout our married life, I never tried to get into her belief system. She was raised in a house filled with Catholic icons like, crucifixes in every room, a statue of the Virgin Mary, a stone statue of St. Anthony in the yard. It was part of her culture, a part of her heritage.

Florence often shared stories with me about growing up Catholic. She still can name a nun or two. One in particular was her third-grade teacher, Sister Regis. She is the one who made her hold her nose to the blackboard because she didn't do her homework.

The nuns wanted to ensure that Florence's soul would be saved. They made her memorize prayers. They stressed how important the sacraments were. To Florence, guardian angels were real, and everyone had one. Souls in purgatory would finally be released, and there are saints we could talk to, especially St. Anthony, patron saint of lost things. She learned that evil existed and was very real. But more than that she understood that real prayer would invoke the graces from God, offering protection from the evil that surrounds all of us. Like Florence, my relationship with God was very real, but I don't think I knew how to pray. I found myself growing more and more distant, feeling detached from the church laws I had been taught. Florence never was detached and never lost her intimacy with the church. The struggles I faced were mine, and it was a sensitive topic that I would not share with her or anyone. But I indeed admired her for her devotion to her Catholic upbringing. Maybe, I had known all along her beliefs and took them for granted, as I did my own Catholic heritage.

In Florence's Own Words

"October 5th – 10th: Had to go get a shot to raise White Blood Count (WBC). So far so good! Been extremely lazy. Get up to move around and get tired very quickly. Had upset stomach past few days. My stomach has been huge since treatment. Can't button any of my pants. Tomorrow I go get Herceptin treatment. I'll ask about stomach when I get there. My head has been pretty sensitive in certain areas, but still have hair on it. Maybe the nerve endings are dying already.

October 11th: Herceptin treatment 10:00 AM today. Went and met with Dr. Shroff first then went in for treatment. I told Dr. Shroff my symptoms of a lot of gas, bloating, backache and heartburn and she said that was all normal. I told her I had only taken one nausea pill and she said maybe I'd be one of the lucky ones. (I'm afraid to get too excited - we'll see what happens down the road). She confirmed that I had a bladder infection and I told her the CIPRO was already working. Guy asked about radiation "mammosite". Mammosite is radiation placed into a balloon in the chest area and you leave it in for 5 days and your done. I would need the balloon implant to do this. But its five days in a row two times a day, rather than everyday (except weekends) for six weeks.

October 12th - 14th: Feeling well so far. Just didn't sleep very well last night and I still feel wide-awake today. Hope I sleep tonight. Saturday the 13th I had severe chest pains on and off while we were at Amanda's soccer game. Had to leave and went home and took Maalox. It went away pretty quickly after that. It was pretty scary because there was no heartburn, just constant pain in the front and back of my chest. I had white pizza for lunch with roasted tomatoes on it. I think the tomatoes may have caused it.

October 15th - 17th: Been getting bloody nose's for past few days. Not bad, just on and off during the day. Also my left eye has been draining a little gooey stuff. Got stuff to put in nose so it wouldn't dry up and got "refresh" to put in eye. May need something else.

Today (Wed. 17th) went and got Herceptin injection. Got really tired and went home and slept for 2 hours. Otherwise, uneventful! Tomorrow, heading to Georgia with Theresa and Bev. Be back Tuesday 23rd."

Saint Peregrine - The Cancer Saint

I often wonder why many people have a hard time accepting the idea of asking saints to pray for them. Even in my own family, the non-Catholic members, state, "Why do you pray to saints when you can pray directly to God? Others say praying to saints and Mary is wrong and condemned by the Bible.

The Catholic Church has always taught that Catholics are to worship God alone, and that prayers to Mary and the Saints are only prayers asking for their intercession on our behalf, and for me I cannot find any fault in that. I know there is only one mediator between God and me and that person is Jesus Christ. However, I do value that there are members of my church, members of my family, and many friends, praying for Florence and me, and these examples can be found throughout the Bible. For those who are familiar with St. Paul, he encourages us to pray for each other. Now, for those of you wondering where I'm going with this, well believe it or not, there is a saint we Catholic's pray to. He is the patron Saint of those afflicted with cancer, AIDS and all the sick. His name is St. Peregrine.

[40]He was born in Forli, Italy around 1265. St. Peregrine dedicated himself to the sick, and the poor. He imposed a special penance on himself to stand whenever it was not necessary to sit. This led to varicose veins. The varicose veins deteriorated into an open, running sore on his leg. The open, running sore was diagnosed as cancer. The wound became so obvious, odorous and painful that the local surgeon scheduled surgery to amputate the leg.

[41]St. Peregrine was confronted with the ugliness and suffering of his own life. At the age of sixty he was challenged to carry a new and more difficult cross. [42]The night before the operation he prayed before the image of the crucified Christ in the priory chapter room. His prayer led him into a deep trance-like sleep during which he envisioned the crucified Christ leaving the cross and touching his cancerous leg. When Peregrine awakened he discovered the wound healed and the leg was saved.

St. Peregrine lived 20 more years. He died on May 1, 1345 at the age of eighty. [40]He was canonized on December 27, 1726. He has been named the Patron Saint for those who suffer from cancer. His feast day is celebrated on May 4th.

I'm Learning How to Pray

"If you remain in Me and My words remain in you, ask for whatever you want and it will be done for you."
John 15:7

"Ask for whatever you want and it will be done for you." That's what it says. That should be easy. I should be able to ask for anything, like removing any threats of cancer from Florence. The problem is it doesn't work that way, because if it did, we would have peace in this world; hatred would be removed from men's hearts, and we would have cancer cures, and so on, and so on. The answer to the problem is in the words above, "Remain in Me and my words remain in you." I believe Our Lord is telling me to stay with Him, do not give up, and trust Him. Once I'm able to achieve that relationship, and His words remain in me, only then can I turn to Him for His help. I sincerely believe this, but first I need to solve some fundamental problems. I needed to deal with my own unfaithfulness, my fear, my confusion, my sinfulness, and the nagging doubts of my beliefs.

To start I need to maintain a mental focus when I try to pray. Often, I find myself thinking about other things or even daydreaming instead of talking to God. I need a small amount of quiet time each day if I'm to practice a sense of spirituality while I try to pray. However, to find a quiet place has been difficult for me. I'm told we can find God in all the usual tasks of our daily life, and if I try to pay attention I can find him there. But, what I'm really seeking is a quiet time, a place where I can turn to God and learn how to pray to Him, and then ask Him for His help.

While attending a class about the life of St. Paul, I read in Rom 8:26,

"The [43] Spirit helps us in our weakness; for we do not know how to pray as we ought, but the Spirit himself intercedes with sighs too deep for words."

"I believe; help my unbelief!"
Mk 9:24

A wonderful prayer of the sick child's father, in the Gospel of Mark! To repeat – "I believe; help my unbelief!"

There is so much to learn when reading scriptures. "Turn to God as you learn how to pray" our church teaches. There are so many examples out there for me. It should be easy for me to learn how to pray.

The Thesaurus defines praying as invoking, and/or communicating with God, worshipping, begging, and pleading. It associates prayer with devotions, services, and petition. [44]The church says, "few sincere words from the heart are more pleasing to God than a large number of repeated devotions, prayers or words." But the church also says, "when appealing to God for favors, it is essential to have a sound faith. [44]Those who believe that God will answer their prayers because they were baptized and married in the Catholic Church, but who never go to Church on Sunday, do not have a sound faith. Their religion is artificial; they are Catholics in name only." Are they talking about me?

By my own admission, my faith has never been valid. As I reflect on my life now, I recognize more than ever, God has given me many opportunities. The door has always been open for me, and yet so many times I did not enter, missing so many of those opportunities. Looking back at my life, missed opportunities are the biggest regrets I have. My spiritual growth should have never been about my personal opinion of what religion should be, but on the contrary, should have been through my association with the Body of Christ. "Faith without actions is dead."

Today, I am enjoying a relationship with God, and now more than ever, I find it necessary to call on Him, to speak to Him and to listen to Him. [44]Yes, to listen to Him. There is a time to talk and there is a time to listen. If I do all the talking, when will I ever hear God speaking to me in my heart? When will I ever hear the inner voice of the Holy Spirit who seeks to guide me in all things?

Now that Florence has completed her first chemotherapy treatment we will await the expected and the unexpected, and the life threatening, dreaded side effects if indeed they come. Yes, I need God's help now, and yes I will pray to Him, - I will speak to Him. I will not miss this opportunity.

The Dreaded Side Effects

The nausea did start, forty-eight hours later along with back pain. For the next five days, Florence will spend most of the time in bed. Her eating habits changed considerably. There were foods she usually enjoyed in the past, but now she could not think about, let alone try to eat them. Some foods were metallic in taste, and then there were some she wanted to have but could not because it would invoke stomach cramps.

When we first formed the medical team we also added a nutritionist. The first meeting was extremely valuable, as we would learn later. We discussed the different foods that could cause problems for Florence. It would be necessary for her to eat something before receiving her treatments. A light meal or snack before her chemotherapy treatment would help! They say you get tired while receiving chemotherapy. Fatigue really is a lack of energy, and we were told it is very common during chemotherapy. Florence's nutritionist suggested eating a balanced diet that includes protein meat, milk, eggs, etc., to help boost her energy. Other suggestions to reduce fatigue were to prioritize her activities, doing the most important ones when she has the most energy and to balance rest and activity so that it does not interfere with her nighttime sleep. She also suggested, "Don't be hard on yourself if side effects make it hard to eat. [45]Try eating small, frequent meals or snacks. Go easy on fried or greasy foods. These can be hard to digest. [45]On days when you are feeling well and your appetite is good, try to eat regular meals and snacks. Be sure to drink plenty of water or liquids, eight to ten 8-ounce glasses each day." Later, we will learn how important it was for Florence to stay hydrated.

We both learned so much from that meeting, and there would be a time we would be grateful to have met with a nutritionist.

During the next six days, Florence endured the side effects as best she could. We kept ourselves busy with trips back and forth from the stores, even though we didn't need to be there, it kept her mind off the chemo reactions.

The evenings seem to be the toughest for some reason. Not sure why. Nausea was always there, but she never had to vomit. When the sensations were there, it was short-lived. The other side effect from Chemotherapy was how tired Florence got. It was amazing and somewhat of a surprise to see how fatigued she really got. It was like all of her energy was sapped out of her system. It would be the cause of one of the biggest emotions with which I would have to cope. To walk into her bedroom in the middle of the afternoon, to see her lying in bed asleep, was very difficult for me. Again, the frustration of not being able to fix this problem overwhelms me. As time goes by, and the side effects continue, it will become even more challenging for me.

It seems that, after six days, Florence starts to rebound. Slowly the nausea and the muscle aches subside. Considering all of the events that had taken place Florence and I were pleased with the first treatment cycle, and we both agreed it was not nearly as bad as we had expected.

It didn't take very long for Florence to start losing her hair. Early one morning I had returned from my daily visit at the Chapel and upon entering quietly into the bedroom, I found Florence wide-awake, looking into a mirror. "What's wrong?" I asked. Florence looked at me and said, "It's started, look, my hair is starting to fall out." I wasn't sure how to react upon this inevitable news. I was so very concerned about her and her feelings. She had known all along it would happen, but to wake up one morning and to actually see it happen was a little disheartening to her. I tried to make light of it knowing it would eventually grow back. I also knew Florence's oncologist would give her a prescription for a "cranial prosthesis," a fancy name for a wig. My feeling was she would experiment. Maybe she'll be daring and go with a curly look and different color. It would be her choice.

The research says, "If you are taken chemotherapy, you probably will lose your hair." The general rule is that the hair falls out around fourteen days after the first treatment. It begins as a few strands on the pillow, then clumps in your comb and wads in the shower drain. I didn't tell her that she would probably lose her hair, but also her eyebrows, eyelashes, and other body-hair. No hair anywhere.

Florence's reaction was very brave as she described what had happened. She took it in stride, and mustered a smile and said, "They say bald is beautiful, don't they Guy?" I immediately knew she wanted me to agree and answer her. What do you think I said to her?

Florence may have tried to present a positive attitude toward the hair loss, but I sensed it was distressing and emotionally draining for her. For so many women and men, we look to continue to examine our perception, and so often we don't like what we see. Hair is one of those things that help define our identity, but really, it never mattered to me, and her hair has never been an issue; she was always beautiful.

The next day we visited the American Cancer Society to meet with a cosmetologist who gave Florence great tips on makeup during chemo and samples from many cosmetic manufacturers. She also carried wigs and would style one for Florence while we were there. This was something I always wanted to do, sit and watch Florence get her hair styled. You guys out there know being around women when they're talking about their hair is one of those things that need lots of patience. Emotions seem to invoke laughter and anger about how their hair looks. What I really like about Florence is how she knows how to create a look that is fashionable and compliments her personality. Actually, I did enjoy watching her try different styles of wigs. Oh, well, part of my caretaking, I guess. As she tried one on, she would turn from the mirror and look at me. "What do you think? Do you like it, or should I try the other one?"

This went on for a little while, and finally she found one she liked and of course I gave her the "OK."

The trip to the American Cancer Society seemed to give Florence a big lift, and I was pleased to have been with her. This was one of those infrequent pleasant experiences Florence had, and to see her smile, was very gratifying to me.

Since there is a limited time between chemo treatments, we try to take advantage of the time to keep busy. It was also an opportunity for Florence to visit with her sisters in Atlanta. Although I was hesitant for her to travel, she really wanted to take advantage of the opportunity to be with her sisters. I didn't let her know, but I was concerned that a side effect may occur, and I wouldn't be there for her. Since her initial diagnosis, I had never left her side. This would be the first time, and she would be some 600 miles away. However, if she had to be gone, she would at least be with her sisters whom I trust so very much.

October 18th - Florence Visits Her Sisters in Atlanta

Florence has been blessed to have brothers and sisters who have a deep sense of love, loyalty for, and devotion to each other. I thank God for blessing her with sisters and brothers that throughout Florence's ordeal kept her smile intact. However, there is a very unique bond that Florence and her sisters have which is, unlike her brothers. The three sisters throughout the many years continue to share their little secrets, their joys, and their wonderful successes as only sisters can do. I continue to respect and admire her sisters in the face of Florence's diagnosis. Many relationships come and go, but this one will last forever.

"A sister is a gift to the heart, a friend to the spirit, a golden thread to the meaning of life."
- Isadora James

Florence loves being with her sisters. She was the second oldest sister and always enjoys the long conversations and the honest sharing with them. There is an unexplainable joy and excitement just being with them, yet no three women could be so different. Theresa, the youngest, has the look of a businesswoman. She has worked most of her adult life and has raised four wonderful children along with her husband Frank. She loves being with all the family at any time. Beverly, the oldest, was the maternal homemaker. Although she worked at her local police department, her favorite pastimes are creating crafts and taking care of her grandchildren along with her husband, Ken. Beverly is easygoing, completely candid, and loves participating in the family parties. The family can always count on her to design decorations for whatever occasions come up.

My observations, when I had the opportunity to be with them, was the wonderful bond among the three of them that did not require any common interests or even similar personalities. Their bond was based on love of family, a shared heritage from their mom and dad. They shared stories of their childhood and growing up together. They laughed. They cried together. Their love was contagious to anyone around them and was rooted in who they were: They were sisters. They were sisters whose love and commitment to each other saw them through life's challenges and joys. Watching Theresa and Beverly around Florence was inspirational, to say the least. It was easy to feel the love they had for her during her cancer journey, especially her dealing with chemotherapy.

When Florence returned from her trip, she was elated and excited about her visit with her sisters. It made me feel so good about how she was feeling. All of the concerns I had before she left seemed to be an overreaction to my caretaking duties. It was a lesson, again; I learned about her being the team leader. On the way home from the airport, she continued telling me stories about her visit. She described to me the morning she went in to take a shower. She began brushing her hair and noticed globs of it on the brush. The chemo was really working! She called her sisters and showed it to them. Their reaction, she said, was somewhat funny to her. Both of their eyes got huge. They didn't know how to react. They didn't want to cry and upset her. But Florence started laughing, and then all three of them started to cry, and then they all laughed again. This broke the ice. As they laughed, each offered in their own way alternative hair suggestions. I thought to myself, "What hair"? I can't imagine why women go through, all the time and trouble, and the money they spend on their hair. But, having her sisters around her made her feel so much more confident in dealing with these new distressing side effects of chemo treatments.

I've watched the sisters interact with Florence. I found them to be incredibly good and kind to her. I can't tell you how appreciative I am for Florence having two wonderful and close sisters who continue to bring happiness and love to her. She always talks about them with admiration and love. I will always be grateful to them for all the kindness they've given and continue to give Florence. God bless them both.

In Florence's Own Words

"October 18th - 23rd: Left with Theresa and Bev on Thursday to head to Georgia! Theresa drove the whole way. Got there about 8:30 PM. Really had a fun time on the ride there.

Friday when I got up and started brushing my hair, it started to come out in big chunks. I walked out of the bathroom and showed Bev and Theresa, their eyes looked huge. It was kind of funny. I was okay till a few minutes later when another big chunk came out and I started crying. Of course, Bev and Theresa started crying with me. That was good because all of a sudden we started laughing. I am so glad I was with them, they are so great and a huge support. We went to a place called Dahlonega, Ga. south of Helen, Ga. It was really a neat area and we had a lot of fun. Very nice little shops. On the way home we went to the Premier Outlet stores. That was really fun. Picked up some Christmas gifts, etc. Saturday went to Helen. The traffic was horrible from about 3 miles away, so we pulled over at a restaurant we saw and ate and they had a great shop there. Then on to Helen! It was very disappointing. It was "October-fest" and very, very crowded. The shops really changed also. Lots of tee shirts and commercial souvenirs! Walked around and left within an hour. Sunday went to church and to another shopping area where they had "Home Goods" stores, etc. After that we went to the movies to see "Elizabeth". It was very good. Monday took our time hanging out at Theresa's then went back to the Premier Outlets. Tuesday morning Theresa dropped us off at a shuttle bus place to take us to the Metro train. The train took us right to the airport. It was a very easy way to get to airport and Theresa didn't have to drive the rush hour traffic. Bev and I were really tired, but we had a great time. Theresa was wonderful, as always, and we hated to leave her (and, she didn't want us to go). Ken and Guy picked us up and we went to eat with them. Then home. I am so lucky to have the sisters I have. We are very close and I love them so much."

Florence returned from her trip renewed and ready for the fourth Herceptin treatment. Remember, every three weeks she takes both the chemo and the Herceptin treatments and every week she takes only the Herceptin treatment. All together, including the sixth chemo treatments, she will undergo fifty-two Herceptin treatments. Each chemo treatment lasts for three and a half hours and the Herceptin treatment last for one and a half hours.

The fourth Herceptin treatment went well. There seem to be no complications from the treatment. Only forty-eight more to go, Ugh!

The three weeks came and went. Time seemed to move by very quickly. Soon it was time to start the second cycle of chemotherapy.

October 25th - Second Chemo Treatment

It seems we're both starting to learn a routine as we enter the treatment center. We walk to the reception desk, sign in and then sit down in the waiting room. The patients and their loved ones are also sitting, waiting for their turn to be called. Soon a nurse will call one of them and slowly they will walk to the treatment room and begin the treatment process. Some will need assistance as they go through the doors. A short time later Florence is called. It's time for her to begin her second cycle of chemotherapy. I want so badly to hold her hand and tell her how much I love her, but I can't. Emotions swell up inside me and again I hold it inside. I slowly follow her into the room where she sits in the same chemo chair she sat in three weeks ago.

I'm beginning to know some of the nurses. Very carefully, I try not to second-guess them. We seem to become friends, and I feel they are starting to like me. I joke a little with them, being careful not to step over the boundary. I see the same patients, again, at least by sight, each sitting in the same chemo chair he/she was three weeks ago. Some are by themselves and others have family members supporting them, but all wearing the same expression of pain and concern. I often wonder how many patients have no one to assist them; no one to accompany them, no one to comfort them. They come into the treatment center by themselves and leave by themselves. A surprising thirty-six percent of patients report having no caregiver of any kind to turn to for support. They are alone! How sad.

I'm so blessed, and thank God each day for the opportunity He gave me to be able to be by my wife's side throughout her chemotherapy sessions, to be her caretaker. I recognize that this battle with cancer will have a profound impact on Florence and me, and also on our family and loved ones. All of us will struggle with the challenges of coping and adjusting to these life changes, but with prayers we will prevail.

In Florence's Own Words

"Thursday October 25th: Went for three chemical treatments today at 11:15 AM. Saw Dr. Shroff first and everything was good until they did the blood test. My red blood cells were down so I had to get a new shot for that. And then they added a flu shot. Two extras I didn't expect. It took a little over an hour and a half for just the Herceptin drip. It shouldn't have taken that long. I think the nurse who did it didn't get the thing to drip right. Anyway, the other drippings took about three hours, so it was a long day there. The first thing that started was the heartburn. Took my Maalox and it worked and I slept pretty well on and off.

October 26th Friday: Had to go today to get shot to raise White Blood Count (WBC). This time yesterday's treatment was a little more intense. Had a lot of heart palpitations and a high pulse count (anywhere from 94 to 104). Called the doctor and they set up EKG, Echogram, and a chest x-ray. The EKG and chest x-ray came out fine. I'm waiting for the Echogram results.

November 1st: Herceptin Treatment today. Everything went okay. My hair has been coming out continuously since leaving Theresa's and it's pretty much gone except for a very, very thin layer (strings) of hair left in some places. There are a lot of bald areas. Not going to shave it yet, I like it as a little cushion under hats and scarf's."

Iron Man - November 3rd

Our son Clint had entered an Iron Man competition in January 2007, and wanted so much to complete his goal of not only running marathons, but also completing in an Iron Man competition.

Clint ran for two reasons. The first and main reason was on behalf of all the children suffering from leukemia; to raise funds for the Leukemia Society to further the support and research of blood related diseases. The second reason was to prove that he could and would do it! He made a commitment to get into the "best shape of his life." A great motivating factor for him was achieving something he had never done before.

He started a successful fundraising campaign. He contacted friends and families and wrote to those friends of theirs who might be interested. Support letters from everywhere were sent to Clint. His friends and family were so helpful and there were many local businesses that pledged money too.

Florence and I were so moved when Clint received a check from our own friends. The grandkids also helped with the fundraising. It's the generosity from those whom you do not know that really made Clint's efforts worthwhile.

Clint trained hard, and at times I thought he would not continue, but each time he told me about the kids with leukemia. He called them his heroes, and said they were suffering much more than he was in training for the marathon. He gradually built up his endurance, and participated in a few races to keep him on track.

The day of his first marathon, Clint was nervous even though he had done all he could in training. He was worried he would not finish the 26.2-mile event. When the gun went off, our emotions really took hold. The last mile was the longest. Florence and I could hear people all around us shouting and cheering for their favorites, and when we saw Clint, tears came to our eyes. We were so proud of what he had achieved for the leukemia heroes and himself. We asked Clint, "Would you do it again?" He answered, "Of course I would."

Clint continued to be very active in the Leukemia Society raising money for his heroes, the Leukemia children. He has run five Disney World marathons, and three 100-mile bike rides in Lake Tahoe. But, there was one more goal - to compete in an Iron Man triathlon.

However, this would not be easy. The Iron Man triathlon requires the participant to swim 2.4 miles, bike 112 miles, and run 26.2 miles, a total of 140.6 miles without stopping.

Why a triathlon? To Clint it was another challenge. His enthusiasm and his insistence were enough for him to sign up for the Iron Man triathlon in Panama City Beach, Florida, in January. He would need to be ready for the start of the event November 3rd. Eleven months to train.

The training was rigorous and took time away from his family. Although the family was supportive, it was difficult for them throughout the training period. In the height of training, he was spending Saturdays and Sundays on the roads and in the water. As expected, his forty-four year old body responded to the training. He was surprised at how brutally hard it was to run after swimming and biking.

On July 3rd, his mom was diagnosed with breast cancer. This was devastating news to him, so he dedicated the triathlon, the Iron Man, to her. It was an emotional moment for him and Florence when he told her he would write her name on his leg dedicating his participation in the Iron Man to her.

The challenge was enormous, and Clint had plenty of second thoughts. "Could I really do this?" he said. Although I was worried it would be difficult for him, I felt it was right and knew he would be successful.

In Clint's Own Words:

"I think I'm ready? I moved down to the beach to the start of the swim event. Where is my support group? I cannot find anyone. The outside temperature is 55°. The water temperature is 70°, and seas are flat. The news helicopter flies over head; the national anthem is sung, and at 6:50 AM, the pros are in the water. Still, I see no sign of my support team, starting to worry.

Then just about two minutes before the event starts I see them all. Mom looks as if she is going to cry. I show her the ribbon and her name on my leg, and she starts bawling. This starts a chain reaction with my support team and others near by who were watching. I have only a minute before I swim and I cannot breathe. Oh my God, I'm going to drown in the first fifty yards because I'm crying and I cannot breathe. I had to turn and face the water and relax.

I was able to calm down. I turned around, gave my wife Vickie a kiss, and said "See you at the finish . . ."
Clint

Florence and I had planned to be at the start of the event to see Clint, and give him our support. However, it was not easy to get near him, as there were some 2200 other participants, including thousands of supporters. The swim was to start at 7:00 AM and we were not having any luck in finding him. This upset Florence, as she really wanted to see him. Within a few minutes before the start of the swim, out of this massive crowd we saw Clint's family waving at us. We quickly worked our way to them and saw Clint on the other side of the spectators' fence. The emotions were overwhelming as Clint saw his mom; he turned around and uncovered the wet suit from his leg, exposing the words "For Mom" written there. Florence with tears in her eyes tried to make her way through the crowd. The spectators sensing this very emotional moment opened a pathway for her as she pressed ahead to be with Clint. My grandson said later, "It was like the parting of the Red Sea, grandpa." Clint made his way to the fence and they hugged each other. The spectators around them were also in tears. What an emotional moment it was.

In Florence's Own Words

"Saturday November 3rd: THE BIG DAY!!! Clint, I can't believe your doing this! It started off with the two and a half mile swim in the ocean. Unbelievable. I just couldn't believe Clint was doing this. When Guy and I got to the beach we couldn't find him, but just before they started I saw Vickie and Josh and then Clint just getting ready to go. I started crying because I thought I had missed him and I wanted to see him before he started. When I started crying, the people in front of us stood aside and let me go to the front of the rope, between us, and the swimmers. Clint lifted up his wet suit pant leg and it said "for Mom" with a pink ribbon drawn around it. He came over and I got to hug him and tell him I loved him. It made my day. I would

have been so upset if I hadn't done that. He told me he was doing this for me. WOW!!! How lucky am I? After the swim, he did the 112-mile bike ride and then the 26.2 run marathon. I knew he would finish without a doubt, but I couldn't wait for it to be over. I just wanted to know he was okay. He was, in fact, more than okay, he looked great. He said he got a little sick to his stomach towards the end. But, what helped him was Vickie met him at about the last 30 yards or so and ran with him till just before the finish line. He ran through that ribbon and crossed the finish line. We were all there waiting for him. Of course I couldn't hold the tears back again, but just looking at him knowing he did this (and for me) was overwhelming. I am so incredibly blessed and I thank God for it everyday.

Katie and David Baldwin were at the event with us. David, an officer for the Bay County Sheriffs office was part of the security for the event. Katie is the daughter of long time friends, Tom and Connie Haney. Tom Haney was Clint's Marathon training coach and was instrumental in custom personal coaching programs, individual coaching sessions, and online coaching for Clint. As a result Clint went on to complete 7-marathons, 5-Century bike rides, 5-Olympic Distance Triathlons, plus Sprint Distance Triathlons, numerous ½ Marathons. "Thank you Tom."

We really enjoyed being with them and their three children. The kids were so good. They had a six-pack of beer for Clint at the end of the race.

It was a more than memorable day. It was so great for Theresa and Frank to be there also. They were such a big support for Clint. Family, it's wonderful!"

Clint's race started well, finishing the swim in one hour and eighteen minutes. The 112-mile bike ride was completed in six hours and five minutes with little or no problems. The hardest part of the race was the 26.2-mile run that was completed in five hours and seventeen minutes. The day was amazing. It was the hardest thing I'm sure he had ever done, both physically and mentally. Clint went on to finish the Iron Man, swimming, biking, and running in thirteen hours and five minutes. It was very emotional as Clint crossed the finish line knowing his mom, family, and friends were there. The whole day meant so much to Florence.

It's about what you want it to be - your own personal fitness and your desire to achieve the goal you set for yourself. At the end of that day, Clint did something that relatively few people have done. It was an unbelievable achievement. He will enjoy this moment for what it means to him, and not what others think it means, especially to those who have never run a marathon, let alone a triathlon! Florence and I will also keep this moment, this precious moment, forever in our hearts. Clint was a true Iron Man that day!

November 7th - Heart Palpitations

There's nothing more terrifying than when your heart suddenly goes into overdrive and you feel powerless to do anything about it. Florence experienced this unwelcome event one evening while watching television. She was uncomfortable and nervous. I immediately took her blood pressure with a monitor I had previously purchased. Her heart rate was 100 plus. A few minutes later I took a second reading and the rate was 93. My first thought, it was linked to the Herceptin, the medication she takes every Thursday. Side effects of Herceptin are heart issues, but I can't say whether Florence's heart fluttering was or was not related to the medications. The next day, Thursday, Florence had her regular infusion of Herceptin and then she had an echogram in the afternoon. Both the EKG (Electrocardiogram) and the Echocardiogram test were negative. The EKG is when they put electrodes on your chest, arms and legs and attach you to a host of wires. This shows the electrical activity in your heart at that exact moment. It can show fast or slow rhythms, old heart attacks or other issues.

An Echocardiogram is just an ultrasound of your heart. They put gel on you and roll a transducer on your chest. The ultrasound is helpful because it can give the doctor a real time view of the heart on a monitor providing him with data whereas an EKG is information based on a split second. Florence will continue to be monitored as she continues her treatments.

So what happened? The doctors believed the palpitations were caused by the chemotherapy and/or the Herceptin treatments, but they can't say for sure. Palpitations are most often caused by stimulants such as caffeine, nicotine, alcohol, or by stress.

[46]Your heart pumps blood through the body continuously in a systematic manner. Blood flows from the top right side of the heart (the right atrium of the heart), and moves down the heart tissue into the lower chambers of the heart, called the ventricles. Heart rhythm changes, or arrhythmias, occur when there is a disruption in the heart's normal electrical system, causing it to beat irregularly.

I now add another concern to my growing list. I pray it will not be a serious issue and will not cause any delays in her treatments.

In Florence's Own Words

November 8th: Had Herceptin Treatment today. When they did the blood test my red blood cells were down lower than last time so I got another shot for that. I thought I was just tired from Clint's Iron Man Event, but apparently it was the low red blood cells. Also had an Echogram today."

November 15th - Third Treatment

Florence is half way to the end of her chemo treatments. She began her third full treatment, and after the next two Thursdays she will finish her third cycle. The fourth cycle starts on December fifth with another full treatment.

For about five days she has to deal with the side effects: nausea, back pains, etc., and dealing with the loss of her hair. Many times she says to me, "Don't look at me," as she places her hand over her head. I don't listen, even though I'm only a private in this battle.

In Florence's Own Words

Thursday November 15th: Three Chemical treatments today! Took the steroids yesterday and was up all night. The worst night ever, as far as sleeping! Usually I can doze off now and then but the last time I looked at the clock it was 4:32 AM and so I figure I fell asleep at about 5 AM, and woke up at 6:30 AM. An hour and a half sleep all night. A few hours after taking the steroids I started to get heartburn, but only took Maalox once just before bed. Today after taking the steroids both times, I got heartburn again. Took Maalox and its working. Had to get another shot today for low red blood cells. This is not uncommon to happen with these treatments.

Friday November 16th: Got shot to raise White Blood Count. Slept well last night, just got up two times and took Maalox once. My face had red rash this morning and felt a little hyper. Went to bed at 9:30 PM and slept till 2:00 AM. Laid awake till about 5:00 AM when I had to get up and take a nausea pill.

Saturday November 17th: Stayed in bed till about 8:30 AM. My neck and face are red and flush this morning and looks swollen, along with my stomach."

Sunday evening, the third day of fighting the side effects, we had a big scare. Florence had an episode of hypotension (abnormally low blood pressure), causing my son to call 911. It didn't take long for the medics to arrive. Within minutes they were in the bedroom surrounding her bed. There were six paramedic's taking blood and a EKG. As it turns out, and thank God again, we did not have to take her to the hospital. She came close to fainting a couple of times and was extremely nauseated. This is a new concern, and again we will need to consult with the doctors. This is the first time an event of this type has occurred. It has indeed scared her, as well as me. Florence and I are finding that after each chemo treatment she takes, the side effects get a little more intense.

In Florence's Own Words

"Sunday November 18th: Not feeling well at all today. Can't eat or drink much. Sunday evening was sitting at Clint & Vickie's kitchen bar with Guy & Clint and just said: "I think I'm starting to feel better". Within thirty seconds after that I had a whiteout. Everything just started to fade away, but guess I didn't really pass out. I just remember getting very limp and Guy saying to Clint "grab her". They picked me up, Guy grabbing my legs and Clint grabbing my shoulders. When they tried to get me through the bedroom door, this whistle sound started coming out of my mouth. Clint said, "Mom, are you okay?" I couldn't answer. I just kept making whistle sounds. I'm thinking they're going to kill me before they get me through the darn door. Before I knew it, I was in bed surrounded by 911 rescue men, at least eight of them. Apparently it was Hypotension. All the other vitals were good. Was much better on Monday and Tuesday, but not the best."

Thanksgiving

In Florence's Own Words

"Wednesday November 21st: Had Herceptin Treatment today. Was not feeling great last night or this morning. Went to my Oncologist, and apparently I was dehydrated. I had to get an IV for fluids. UGH!! I felt much better about an hour after that. I have to try really hard to drink a lot more. Red blood cells were low, but didn't get a shot. Hope the nurse didn't forget the shot."

There isn't a day that Florence does not have something special happen in her life. One of those wonderful days is this year's Thanksgiving. I can't help but notice how each day is special and meaningful. The trees and decorations seemed especially wonderful. The lights are brighter, the carols sound sweeter, and I realize more than ever how important my family and friends are.

For the past six months, Florence has undergone an array of medical procedures. From being diagnosed with breast cancer to lumpectomy surgery, to chemotherapy, nausea, days of incredible fatigue, she still continues to stay positive and in good spirits. Well, not all the time. There are times that have been very challenging for the both of us.

Even though she tries to stay positive throughout this most difficult time in her life, there are times when the emotional strain is too much for her to handle. Thanksgiving day we were getting ready to go to Guy Anthony and Janet's home for the day. As we were walking to the car, I wondered why Florence had stopped, not moving, just staring at me. I walked over to her and saw she was extremely upset. I asked her what was wrong? She burst out crying as I held her in my arms. "I can't do this! It hurts, and I'm so frightened. I'm so tired of being sick everyday. I'm not sure I want to continue with the chemo."

As I said before there would be meltdowns. This was a significant one for the both of us. A major meltdown! How do I handle this? What do I say? Words don't seem to work; I just hold on to her trying to comfort her. This is one of those times I would do anything to trade places with her. Again, frustrated, the thought goes through my mind,

"Damn it, why can't I find a way to fix this?" A few moments had passed, and she said to me, "I'm okay now. I'm okay."

We both walked slowly to the car, saying nothing to each other, yet the both of us understood how difficult this journey is becoming.

We arrived at my son's house, and the grandchildren gave us hugs, wishing us a Happy Thanksgiving. Janet and Vickie, Guy and Clint, had decorated the dinner table beautifully, as they have done so many times. What a wonderful family, I thought to myself. Florence and I are indeed blessed.

I usually don't feel so excited about the holidays. It seems we all have forgotten why we celebrate the holidays. Rushing back and forth from the Mall, concerned about what presents we should buy - and for whomever. I was finding myself not enjoying the holidays as I once did. Not this year. Even though I feel stress as Florence goes through chemotherapy, I enjoy each and every minute and try to do all the special things that we associate with Thanksgiving and Christmas. I think of the wonderful things: the stuffing, the turkey, and all the family I love so very much. Thanksgiving with our children and grandchildren was a joy.

In Florence's Own Words

"Thursday November 22n: Thanksgiving! Was up all last night with cramps and an upset stomach. It lasted until late morning. By lunchtime it had pretty much stopped. Was able to have lunch and thanksgiving dinner."

My visits to the chapel are more intense now as I continue to pray for the end of chemo, and that Florence stays strong; and that all cancer cells, if any, are removed from her body.

Last year I didn't know that there was a tumor growing in Florence's body. This year is so different, so much more to be thankful for. I continue to be reminded of so many good things and so many missed opportunities. I have learned one major lesson: not to take a wonderful marriage and family for granted.

There is, however, one feeling I had over the holidays, one I continue to try to suppress. It is probably on Florence's mind also. Will she continue to do as well as she is doing? After all the treatments, a year from now, will Florence have a recurrence? I won't let these thoughts, although sometimes difficult to suppress, interfere with this wonderful season.

As a cancer husband, there are times that are very difficult for me. I was about to leave Florence to meet the family at church as we do every Sunday. Florence was not able to join us and was in bed. I went over to the bed and gave her a hug and told her I was off to church. Before leaving I stared at her for a brief moment. Seeing her in that condition, pale and fatigued, and for the first time she was not able to attend Mass with the kids and me, was indeed difficult. At church, my sons, their wives, and grandkids all sat in the same pew, the nine of us, with one missing. It was indeed a time to pray.

Chemo Sucks

Yes, indeed it does. My sister, Jocelyn, once said that to Florence in an email, as she described her own battle with cancer. Jocelyn is an 18-year breast cancer survivor and has been a wonderful mentor for Florence as they shared their battles with the chemo side effects. After Florence was diagnosed, Jocelyn sent the following email to her:

"You received the worst news any woman can receive. You will receive all types of well meaning, "drink this, eat this etc." Only YOU can make choices. You will be overwhelmed with good reason. Guy will be with you throughout for all your Dr. appointments. It's very important to have another set of ears. The most important thing to remember is it is not a death sentence. You will prevail. You have a strong, praying family. You will always be in my thoughts and prayers each and everyday. - I love you,"
- Jocelyn

Jocelyn is the oldest in my family of three. My other sister, Andréa Louise, was second in line and I was the third. Andréa died of cancer at the age of fifty-four, leaving five children and a husband behind. Andrea's family, Florence and I, my sister Jocelyn and her husband, my mom and dad and other family and friends, attended the funeral where I gave the eulogy. Not a pleasant day to look out into the audience to see her husband and children and try to say the appropriate words. What a difficult situation to see my mom and dad sitting in the front pew next to their daughter's coffin. How often had we heard about the difficulty of losing your child? It's not supposed to happen that way. Yet, I stood before them trying to comfort my mom and dad in this most difficult time of their lives. Yes, chemo sucks, but so doe's cancer!

There are other great friends and cancer survivors who shared, and continue to share, with Florence their ordeal with this menacing disease. Her good friend, Carolyn, in Stuart, Florida, continues to call her, giving her encouraging words while describing her personal events as she dealt with her own cancer. There are others. Her Mormon friend in American Fork, Utah, who emailed her with this wonderful note:

"When I go to the temple next week, I will put your names on the prayer list. You won't mind if a "zillion" Mormons are praying for you, too.
On a more serious note, I believe that Heavenly Father & Jesus Christ know you, personally, Flo, and they are AWARE of the challenges you/Guy face and

will COMFORT you by the sprit of the Holy Ghost. I can almost feel your strength and faith that all will be well just by your recent comments. I, too, believe that all will be well. As we go through life, there are times when we don't understand why "bad things happen to good people." I have certainly had those thoughts in connection with Josh (even Joni!). But I try to keep in mind that there is a purpose to life and a HIGHER POWER. I know that you have a strong belief in Heavenly Father/God as this HIGHER POWER because we have talked about it. So, we just have to "keep on keepin' on." No matter. So, Flo, just "keep on keepin' on" and it will be okay. You are an "awesome" person & so many of us love you. Take care, mind the doctors & hang in there! I will pray for you often. - Love, again,"
- Diane

And then there's my "bestest" chum who writes:

"Flo, I just read your note. We are all members of the Carbonneau fan club. I'm a charter member and actually I want you to kick a few people out. We are here for you at any time day or night. Prayers are coming but at times they seem too easy, so give us something more to do. I'll handle Guy; a little handholding is coming. I am waiting for my buddy to get back to me with his opinion [pathologist opinion]. He is en route to his California home. The one unmistakable issue to keep in focus is that there have been huge successes made in the treatment of breast cancer in the last few years. You will benefit from all of them. The other is that frame of mind plays a huge role and you are perfectly equipped to handle that. Keep totally positive and you'll walk away from this without a doubt. Now about Samoset, Maine, do you know how to paddle a kayak? Can you pick out a huge rock in a fog? We'll have to see!"
Love, Bob"

In Florence's Own Words

"Friday November 23rd: Good day. Went shopping and then to Guy & Janet's for leftovers. Had an uncomfortable stomach most of the day, but was able to eat a little.

Saturday November 24th:

Slept okay (a little restless), but had to get up because my stomach was upset. Took a Tylenol to get back to sleep.

November 29th Thursday: Herceptin Treatment - Got very tired half way through treatment. That never happened before. My red blood cells were very low again. It was at 8.3 and you can't let it get lower than 8 or you have to have a blood transfusion. They gave me an extra strong shot for it this time. We'll see what happens next week. Last week it was low also but they didn't give me a shot. I'm thinking the nurse forgot to give it to me. Maybe that's why it's so low this time. I hope so. Herceptin definitely causes heartburn. It started on the way home. Guy gave Dr. Shroff his ADX book and she was very excited."

Lady in Black - First Meeting

On November 28th, I had the opportunity to visit the St. Stephen chapel to celebrate in the Mass, as I have done so many times before. Again, it was another wonderful opportunity to become completely occupied with myself. I gave all my energy to concentrating on prayers for my wife. Before the Mass started I would often lean over, close my eyes and ask Florence's angels to wrap their arms around her, to keep her safe from the chemotherapy treatments. I knew who Florence's angels were, so it was easy for me to ask them to intercede and pray for Florence. These wonderful angels were Florence's mom, Florence, my mom Yvette, my sister Andréa, and our sister-in-law, Barbara Jo Hyland. There were others: my dad, her dad and so many more loved ones who have left this world and whom I would also ask to intercede and pray for her. My mom, my sister, and Barbara Jo knew very well the difficult journey Florence was going through. They too had suffered from this insidious disease - a disease that finally took them away from us.

As I was leaning over, immersed in prayer, I felt a tap on my shoulder that startled me. I turned around to see who it was. A young lady was seated directly behind me, and immediately apologized for interrupting me.

She said, "Guy, I've been here on several Wednesdays and could not help in watching you as you prayed. It seemed to me you were going through a difficult time, and I wondered if I could pray for you."

I was very surprised, not only her knowing my name, but the kindness shown to me.

"Yes, I am going through some tough times."

I continued telling her about Florence and her diagnosis and the chemo treatments she was undergoing.

She responded, "Your wife will get past this and someday she will look back and be amazed, and thankful at all the good things that have happened."

I was simply overwhelmed by the generosity of this incredible lady. I tried to compose myself. I certainly was not going to break down in front of a stranger. What a wonderful and thoughtful person, I thought to myself. If someone is kind enough to take the effort to make you feel good, that person must feel really good about himself or herself. Right now I'm blushing, and wonder what her story is. I ask her, "It seems to me you also may be going through some difficulties?"

She replies, "Yes, well, not really. By the way, my name is Lesley."

"Happy to meet you, Lesley," I said.

With a continuing smile on her face, she explained that she was cancer free since last July. She had lost a lung from the disease and had been going through all the cancer treatments available. I asked her how she was feeling and she responded with great enthusiasm.

"I feel great, wonderful. Even with one lung missing I'm still as active as I always was."

What a wonderful attitude I thought to myself. She needs to meet Florence. They are so much alike. The Mass started, and I thanked her for her concerns and comments.

A couple of weeks had passed when again, visiting the chapel; I felt a tap on my shoulder. I turned, and there was Lesley! We exchanged "hellos," and she immediately asked how Florence was doing. I responded, "She's doing okay," with a little hesitancy. "Chemo is tough for her."

"Guy," she said. "All of this will pass, and she will be fine." She reaches over and carefully pulled out a blanket.

"Please give this blanket and this note to your wife. It is a "cancer blanket" and I want her to have it. It will keep her warm during her chemo treatments."

I was really caught off guard with this one. Immediately I had a lump in my throat and a tear in my eye.

"Lesley," I said. I was speechless. All I could say was, "Thank you."

I brought home the blanket and the note, woke up Florence and told her the story of how I first met Lesley two-weeks ago and now, this morning, the blanket. Florence was very curious and said, "Why would a perfect stranger start a conversation, know your name, and then give you a cancer blanket to give to me?"

"Don't know," I said. "She probably got my name from Fr. George. She did tell me she knew him." Florence opened the note and read it to me. It said:

"Dear Florence,

Just wanted to let you know that so many people are thinking good thoughts for you everyday - even people you don't know. I wanted to give you this little poem my daughter gave to me one day. She thought I looked sad.

Florence, I promise you the love around you will carry you through this time. You will look back at a later date and feel so thankful and yet amazed.

Sending you loads of happy, healthy and loving thoughts,
- Lesley"

"Angels fly here and there, angels stop by everywhere.

Angels give you blessings, if they hear you have been confessing when you have done something wrong.

Angels go to every place, and flying around in dresses made of lace and let people know that they are loved. So just remember if you are feeling sad or blue, remember how many people love you.
- Alexa"

With tears in her eyes Florence said, "What a special person. I would really love to meet her."

December 4th - Shingles

Florence had finished the third cycle of chemotherapy. She was half way, and the next week she would begin her fourth of six cycles of treatments. Normally every Thursday of every week is when she is scheduled to take the treatments, however, because of a scheduled family Christmas party she asked to be treated a day earlier so she could attend the celebration and be with her brothers and sisters. Before the Christmas party, Florence was recovering from her Herceptin treatment over the weekend. Sometime on Sunday she started to experience back pains. In the past, she had similar pains and attributed it to her injections of Aranesp, used to treat low red blood cell counts or anemia. But this time it was different.

The pain persisted through Monday. It was then that I looked at her back and noticed various blotches of redness located on the middle of her back and to the right. Each patch had a different degree of redness and size, the largest the size of a quarter. What was this, I thought? I have read most, if not all, of the side effects, and this was not mentioned in any of the documentation. I reread the clinical data on Taxotere, Carboplatin and Herceptin, the treatment protocol she was taking, and found no mention of anything like this. Again, I'm overwhelmed with emotions, feelings I cannot let Florence see. I needed to step back and step into my analytical world. I don't know anything about this! I don't know anything about cancer! I have to quit thinking I can fix everything. I can't fix this. I look at Florence's saddened face, a face I've seen so many times now. I said to her, "I'll call your GP and schedule an appointment for you right away. Try not to worry its probably just some kind of rash or something! He'll give you some medicine to fix it."

In Florence's Own Words

"I had a little itch under my right left back shoulder (around wing area) for a few days and then I started having a pain in what felt like my muscle there. I had a little red mark there. I watched it for a couple of days thinking something may have bit me. But, it continued to get more painful, very itchy

and there are now three or four welts all around that area. Yesterday and especially last night it was very painful and I did not sleep much at all the past few days."

"Shingles," I said, in anger, "Why would she get Shingles in the middle of chemotherapy?"

The doctor understanding my concern said, "It happens. Over age sixty, about ten percent will have a Shingles episode. Because of Florence's immune system being compromised from her chemo treatments, she was at risk."

"What now?" I asked, still angry.

"We'll treat her with Valtrex, and I'll give your oncologist my diagnosis."

In Florence's Own Words

"Today I am going to see Dr. Kovats. Bad news. I have shingles. Dr. Kovats took one look at my back and the first thing he said was "oh no". I didn't say a thing. Then he said "oh you poor thing, wow". Guy and I just looked at each other and he confirmed what Guy thought it was, Shingles. I think I felt more sorry for Guy at the time than me. He looked devastated. He got upset and said: "How could this have happened?" I really felt bad for him. On the way home he didn't say much and looked very upset. I said a little prayer for him. My treatment tomorrow is cancelled."

It was time again to go back to my research mode and find out what Shingles is and what Florence would be in for. My sister Jocelyn told me she had Shingles three weeks before starting her chemotherapy. It was not pleasant, and the pain was the greatest factor she had to contend with.

Shingles can be a serious threat to life in an immune suppressed person. Since Florence is taking chemotherapy the treatments, unfortunately, had damaged the good cells that usually fight invading organisms. Now that Florence has been diagnosed with Shingles, there is a possibility that the virus will spread throughout her body, reaching vital organs like the lungs, causing viral pneumonia or secondary bacterial infection.

The viral infection caused by the varicella zoster virus, is a common disease among children. We know it as chickenpox. The issue is when the chickenpox rash heals, the virus remains in the nervous system of the affected individual in a dormant state for years. Later, usually after age sixty, if the individual's immune system is weakened, the virus can be reactivated and shingles can appear. This apparently is what happened to Florence. I continued to research Shingles and found a very disturbing side effect. Shingles can lead to long-term, painful conditions after the rash and blisters have healed, called Post Herpetic Neuralgia (PHN), nerve pain that persists after the rash is gone. About twenty percent of people with Shingles develop PHN. Florence already has back pains causing me to worry about what she will be facing.

I immediately called Florence's oncologist and gave her the diagnosis. The oncologist had already heard the report from Florence's doctor and canceled all her treatments. Until the Shingles had run its course, it would not be wise to continue treatments. In most people, this rash typically disappears within three to five weeks, but the pain may last forever. If we caught the signs of Shingles early enough, within seventy-two hours of onset, we can start an antiviral medication such as Valtrex that should significantly reduce the duration of the symptoms. This will help speed healing and reduce the risk of developing complications such as Post Herpetic Neuralgia. If, in fact, Florence does well and the Shingles dry up, she could continue her treatments sometime in late December.

The unwelcome news was depressing for both of us. It is the first time I felt real anger and could not accept that she had Shingles. All the side effects from chemotherapy, I understood, but Shingles? We were looking forward to the last chemo treatment in early January, but now Florence would have to deal with this unwanted scourge and the pain associated with Shingles. Would she be one of the twenty percent who will have to deal with Post Herpetic Neuralgia? Who knows!

Each year, one million Americans develop Shingles. Approximately ten percent of adults will get Shingles at some point during their lifetime, usually after the age of fifty. The good news is that most people do not get shingles more than once because they develop immunity to the virus. However, about [47]one percent to five percent of individuals will suffer a recurrence of shingles either in the original area on the body or a different area. Individuals may be most susceptible to recurrent attacks when they are run down or have a weakened immune system.

The treatment for Shingles is VALTREX. This anti-herpetic medication is widely used in the treatment of shingles. This was the drug of choice the doctor prescribed for Florence. VALTREX is proven to speed healing, reduce the pain, and keep new blisters from forming. VALTREX works to help stop the varicella-zoster virus from multiplying. The medication needs to be used early in the course of shingles, within two or three days of the rash. Florence and I believed we were well within the 72 hours since the pain first started. It is very possible that Florence may be rid of this within the next two weeks or so. I pray this be the case. VALTREX, however, does not lessen the pain. She will be preoccupied with unrelenting pain until it finally goes away.

In Florence's Own Words

"Wednesday December 5th: The pain in my back is much worse. And, the welts are coming out more.

December 6th- 7th: This is not fun. The pain is bad and I had to take 2 pain pills instead of one."

It is not only the pain she will have to deal with, but also she will need to be concerned with the possibility her Shingles is contagious to anyone who has not had chickenpox. Research shows a person with Shingles can pass the virus to individuals who have never had chickenpox, and if they are infected, they will develop chickenpox - not Shingles. However, a person with chickenpox cannot communicate Shingles to someone else. For anyone to develop Shingles, he/she must already harbor the virus in the nervous system. Anyone who does harbor the virus, having contact with someone with chickenpox will not trigger Shingles. And, finally, a person with Shingles cannot transfer Shingles to someone else.

I have said I visited each morning the chapel at St. Stephen, and it is there that I find solace and faith that Florence will get through all of this. It continues to be a place that provides comfort in times of sadness and disappointment. And one can only imagine my disappointment knowing Florence had Shingles to contend with now. There is a cancer prayer I learned early on and want to share it with you, the reader . . .

"I pray for my faith in God, the Great Physician, will give Florence and me - hope.

Father, [48]You have written in Your Word "How God anointed Jesus of Nazareth with the [48]Holy Spirit and with power: who went about doing good, and healing all who were oppressed of the devil; for God was with Him." God, please send an anointed servant to lay hands on my wife Florence and let her recover in Jesus's Mighty Name. Father, I curse the root cause of this disease and declare that Your healing virtue flows through Florence, in Jesus's Powerful Name, Amen."

December 8th - Family Christmas Party

Slowly, Florence is responding to the Valtrex medication, and the pain seems to be subsiding. She felt well enough to attend a family Christmas party at her brother's home in St. Petersburg, Florida. I was cautiously excited for her to be able to be there with her brothers and sisters and their spouses. Although she was fatigued at times, and there were a few episodes of nausea and pain, she handled the setbacks like the trouper she is. There was one incident where she was asking for something cold, sweet, and soft to eat. Ice Cream! Not good as it turns out. Sometime later she started to get nauseated, and for the next six hours, she had to deal with that sick feeling in the pit of her stomach and the dreaded urge to vomit. Her body is telling her something is wrong inside, but she can't do anything about it. She had to lie down with the hope the symptoms would pass. I felt sorry for her. I found out later that taking any dairy products is a "no-no" when taking VALTREX. It wasn't until the next morning that she felt better.

In spite of some setbacks, I doubt anything would have held her back from being with her brothers and sisters. All of them tried to help or to offer suggestions making her as comfortable as they could. In retrospect, it was a good weekend.

In Florence's Own Words

"Thursday December 6th: Left to visit my brother Jim and his wife, Joy for a Family Christmas party. My other brothers and sisters also came with their spouses. Thursday and Friday wasn't good for me. Last night I got very sick, felt terrible. This morning when I got up, I joined everybody for breakfast. They all were almost done, but they sat with me and we talked and had fun conversations. When I was done, I started to head to the family room and got very nauseated, and very light headed. I made it to the couch and put my feet up. Felt a tiny bit better, but not great. Guy got me some of my nausea pills, which helped a little. The family all went out in the boat to get lunch. I was really disappointed I couldn't go; it was such a beautiful day. I just did not feel well at all. They are all so great; they waved at me as they left. It really made me feel good. Of course, my unbelievable, wonderful husband stayed with me. We stayed out on Jim's patio and watched them till we couldn't see them anymore. Jim and Joy have the most beautiful place, so

it wasn't all that hard to stay home. We saw some dolphins in front of their dock while we were out there, so beautiful.

December 8th: Saturday was the family Christmas party and all the family came. It was great. We took a ride in the boat in the evening to see the boat parade. It was so pretty. The neat part was there were several dolphins that were riding the waves. The kids loved it. A memorable part of the ride was when Skyler, eight years old, came over to me, put her arms around me and asked: "How are you doing Aunt Florence?" I said I was doing pretty well, and she replied "That's good because I pray for you every night". Talk about how great this whole family is, even the little ones. Anyway, really had a good time, and a lot of fun. So much love and support this whole weekend. Jim and Joy were great hosts the whole four day stay."

His Holiness the Dalai Lama said,
"This is my simple religion; it is the philosophy of kindness."

The following week, December 12th, I met Lesley in the chapel. She, in her kind way, asked how Florence was doing. "She's doing fine," I said, "Can't wait for her to finish the chemo treatments." Again, exactly like the weeks before, she reaches down and grabs a decorated bag filled with gifts.

"Please," she says, "Give this to Florence. I know she will enjoy them."

"Lesley," I said, "You have to stop doing this."

"Oh Guy, its nothing, besides she will use the items in the bag."

"Thanks Lesley. Is there anyway you could join us for coffee some morning? Florence would love to meet you."

"Yes, I would love to," she said.

During the Mass that morning I thought about what she had said to me. About her cancer, her family, and her husband and how she coped with her cancer. I felt there were other things going on with her. There was a hint that maybe there was a recurrence, although she never said so. I worry about her and pray for her.

In Florence's Own Words

"December 11th: Had two full nights of insomnia. Called doctor and she said it was normal, and prescribed Ambien for sleeping. Hopefully it works."

December 13th - Florence Starts Her Fourth Treatment Cycle

Florence's battle with Shingles seems to be over. The pain she had endured has drastically subsided, and except for some itching now and then, we both think it's gone. Because of the Shingles episode, today's treatment was only to include the infusion of Herceptin and not the chemo drugs, Texotere and Carboplatin. However, after meeting with the oncologist it was decided that she start today with the full treatment again. Florence and I did not expect this to happen. We knew that because of Shingles, delaying the treatments was inevitable since her immune system had been compromised. However, Dr. Shroff and Dr. Kovats felt she was over the Shingles, and it was important for her to get back on her treatment schedule. Florence and I looked at each other, wanting for one or the other to make the decision to continue with the treatment. This was not my decision. It was Florence's. Deep down I wanted her to continue, but it was her decision. Again, the team leader was quiet. Staring at the floor, and then moving her eyes toward me, she said, "Ok Dr. Shroff, lets move ahead." For many reasons it was better that Florence agreed to move forward. The downside is she will have to cope with the side effects for the next five to seven days. The good side is Chemo will stop on January 24th instead of February 28th. The next full treatment is January 3rd, the fifth cycle, if all goes well.

In Florence's Own Words

"Three chemical Treatments. Thought I was getting Herceptin treatment only today because of shingles, but Dr. Shroff thought I was well enough to do the three-chemical treatments (she had postponed this till the 27th). I was glad because now I only have two more of these to go. January 24th should be last one. Can't wait!! Had to take two Ambien's to sleep. The first one didn't work and it took over an hour for the second one to work, but finally slept. Thank you God!!

December 14th Friday: Had bone marrow shot today for white blood cells. These hurt!"

So, Florence took the treatment today knowing there are only two more to go. Yes, she probably will have some difficulty the next seven days but then it starts to get better for her. We are hopeful she will have a great Christmas with the family.

In Florence's Own Words

"Saturday December 15th: Not the best day. Slept on and off last night, only took one sleeping pill, probably should have taken two. I was okay in the morning, went to do a little shopping for about an hour and a half. When I came home I didn't feel good. Lay around most of the day. My legs were jumping quite a bit before I went to bed. Took 2 sleeping pills, I NEED TO SLEEP.

Sunday December 16th: Slept six and a half hours last night, it was great, first time in four days. So far so good this morning!

Monday December 17th: Went to Guy & Janet's for dinner. Ate a little bit of everything she had, but shouldn't have. Was up till about 2:00 AM with my stomach aching. I thought I was going to bring it all up but I took a nausea pill, which worked. Slept okay the rest of the night and woke up about 9:30 AM."

For the last six months Florence has been on a journey; one she did not want to take, but one she had to take. The journey has been on a rough road with many hills for her to climb, but she was able to climb each one. Although the road may have been bumpy, there were planned rest stops along the way, one of which is coming up this Tuesday. The timing couldn't be better for her, and she is looking forward, as I am, to celebrating the holidays with our sons, their wives, and our wonderful grandchildren.

In Florence's Own Words

"December 25th: Merry Christmas! Going through this during the holidays has been really good. I've been busy and haven't had a lot of time to think about anything else. Had a wonderful Christmas, as usual. The kids and grandkids are so great. I'm so thankful and blessed to have Guy

and them. They are all so caring, especially Amanda. She is an angel. She is always holding my hand, or sitting next to me and making sure I'm okay, asking if I need, water, food, or anything? She is pretty amazing."

She and I have been incredibly blessed all along this trip with the support and love from all of our family and friends. The emails continue to come from everywhere, and many contain the same message. "We have you in our prayers." I cannot tell you how much this has meant to Florence and me. It is the reason her road has been less difficult to travel on and the hills easier to climb.

The best metaphor I can think of is,

"Life is like a river. It's easier to let the current carry you than it is to swim against it. This does not mean that it is an effortless ride. Parts of the river will be hazardous, requiring great skill to navigate safely."

Shortly after Christmas, Florence will finish her 5th cycle of chemo treatments, leaving only two more treatments to go. But, her journey does not end there. Approximately two weeks after the end of her chemo treatments she will start radiation treatments, once every day for six weeks.

Her journey continues, but what helps to make it a little easier is our family and friends with her on her journey.

In Florence's Own Words

"During one of my treatments I sat next to a girl who looked like she was in her late forties. Her husband walked in with her and as soon as he left the room she started crying. I leaned over and put my hand on her arm and asked if this was her first day of treatment. It was. I felt so sorry for her. She did the same thing I did on my first day of treatments. She was so scared. I talked to her for a few minutes and between wiping her eyes and nose, and me trying to hold back my tears, we both started laughing. I guess the emotions just struck us funny. Anyway, she had quite a sad story. Her first husband died about 8 years ago and a few years after that she met someone and they married. His first wife died also. They were only married a couple of years and she found out she had a heart problem. She had surgery (not exactly sure what kind)

but continued having problems with her heart up until about two years ago when she finally got a clean bill of health. So when they found out she now had breast cancer, they were quite upset. Her breast cancer sounded much the same as mine and she was going to have the same treatments I was having. I never saw her again because after the day I met her she would be going for her treatments in the Orlando office (I was getting mine in Winter Park office). I would love to see her again someday, but probably very unlikely. I'd just like to know how she is doing and how her treatments were for her. I do feel good though about the fact that she had a husband who reminded me of Guy and who was going to be with her every step of the way."

December 18th - Birds and Florence's Wig

Florence and I were visiting the Disney Boardwalk with her sisters and brothers-in-law. While sitting at a table enjoying ice cream, we were watching birds flying around the trees or on the ground, trying to find leftover scraps of food. Without warning, a bird flew over Florence and tried to pick the wig off her head. Of course, the incident instigated comments and laughter. Was the bird trying to build a ready-made nest? What would have been Florence's reaction if the bird actually flown away with her hair? Florence said, "Had he been successful, the bird was well on his way to building a condo."

Florence Meets Lesley

Finally, on February 21, Lesley Harris met my wife for coffee. What a wonderful morning for Florence and Lesley. Even though I was there, I was never able to speak. They talked and talked, about everything, about nothing. They each described the treatments they had been going through, their doctors, and how prayer was such a vital component in their battle against this dreaded disease. The more they talked the more the friendship was building. They were both establishing a unique and wonderful bond. One big reason for this success stems from them each being good listeners, and part of being a good listener, is letting the other person know that you are paying attention.

Dale Carnegie once said,
"It's much easier to become interested in others than it is to convince them to be interested in you."

These two gals got it right. Unlike me, they know how to relate, each taking a turn to listen, each taking a turn to speak, or to respond. Boy, so much to learn, as my mother would say.

This incredible angel continues to bless Florence with a wonderful friendship. They continue to meet for coffee, and both of them continue to share their little stories, as well as conversations about the most arbitrary stuff.

Why are humans, when they want to be, so nice to each other? Why are we willing to cooperate with people whom we barely know? I think people do nice acts because it feels good to do it. Isn't that a good thing?

"Humble yourself before others and you will be exalted, and Treat others as you would want to be treated yourself."

Would I have said this if I didn't get my wake-up call back in July when Florence was first diagnosed? I wonder?

The Donut Man

Every week I've been taking Florence to the cancer treatment center, and each time a man would arrive with a box of donuts. I call him the donut man since I never did get his real name. I asked a chemotherapy technician why was he delivering donuts to the center and taking the time to hand them out to each patient, including my wife?

"The donut man knows how to put a smile on the patients faces," the technician said, "as well as putting a smile on your wife's face. He tells the patients they have to smile back at him before he leaves. That's how they 'pay' me," he says."

"So, what's his story?" I asked.

She said, "He once sat in one of those chemo-chairs for several weeks of treatments. After he was through he promised, he would come back to thank all of the technicians and nurses."

"What type of cancer did he have?"

"Don't know," she replied. "But he did come back and has been delivering donuts every week."

I bet many of you readers do not know there is a National Doughnut Day. It's celebrated on the first Friday of June every year. The holiday celebrates the doughnut, a ring-shaped piece of dough, deep-fried and sweetened. I looked this up after watching our donut man's visits to the center.

Why donuts, I thought? I know our brains are programmed to leap into action when presented with sugary treats, such as donuts. It started me thinking that many people really don't know what to do or say when someone becomes sick with a similar disease. Maybe giving the donuts to patients offers hope to battling the disease that he, the donut man, was able to overcome. How do you say, "thank you," to caretakers who are willing to help save you from a disease that is slowly taking your life? What can you do for those people who may be giving you the chance to watch your children grow up? Do you think this is the donut man's inspiration?

The giving spirit of people amazes me. People, who for whatever reason take it upon themselves to offer their support, their love and their generosity.

During Florence's fifth treatment, the donut man wasn't there with his box of donuts. We never saw him again. What happened to him, I wonder? Hopefully he understands that he had found a unique way to put smiles on cancer patients during their chemo treatments, and for that we our thankful for his visits - and the donuts. We pray for him, and for his caring generosity.

January 3rd - Fifth Treatment Cycle

Florence has been getting ready for the fifth treatment knowing that there will be at least twelve to fifteen days when she won't be feeling very good at all. It didn't take long to realize this cycle of treatments was not going to be easy for Florence. During previous treatments when Florence walked through the doors of the treatment center I would indicate how many treatments were left by the number of fingers I held up in front of her. After her fifth treatment Florence walked out of the center, slowly, and very pale. In an attempt to cheer her up, I held one finger in the air suggesting there was only one more treatment left. She stared at me and said angrily, "Put the finger down. I doubt seriously I will be here for the last treatment." Oh my, I thought to myself, did I step over the boundary? The day didn't get better.

She spent the rest of the day in bed, totally drained, absolutely no energy. The next day didn't get better either. Nausea, fatigue, and pain haunted her throughout the day. I was so careful not to say anything, only to get her a drink, give her medicine, and just hold her hand. This was a very difficult time for her. It had to be the worst of all the treatments she had taken. We've been aware that chemotherapy side effects are cumulative. It doesn't get better. That's for sure.

As each day went by I wondered if she would be well again. Previously she would start to feel good after the fifth or sixth day. This time was different. It's been over eight days, although she felt a little bit better, she was still struggling with the continuing side effects. However, she got over the effects as the days trudge by.

In Florence's Own Words

"January 3rd: Three chemical treatments: After the treatment we went to a drug store and I got nauseated, my face got very red and I got very bad heartburn. This is the first time I had a reaction so soon. This usually happens next day or two days later. Took a sleeping pill and slept very well. ONLY ONE MORE OF THESE TO GO! YEA!!!!

January 4th: Happy Birthday Guy! I went and had my follow-up shot today (bone marrow - white blood cell) and so far so good, but boy do those darn things hurt. Just feeling a little lethargic today. I think sleeping so well last night really helped.

January 5th: Went to dinner last night for Guy's birthday and didn't do to great. Ate some of a baked potato, but didn't feel good when we left the restaurant or when I got home. Took two Tylenol PM's so I could sleep, but it didn't work well. Took sleeping pill about 2:00 AM and that seemed to work okay. I had a lot of acid reflux and my stomach was upset, so took Maalox and nausea pill. Also had some chills and my legs were jumping, but that didn't last too long. Stayed in bed till almost 11:00 AM. Still not feeling to great. I think Guy had a good time last night. He loves it when we're all together with the kids and grandkids. I do too.

January 6th: Not a good day, very weak, slept most of the day. Got very hot a few times and felt really weak. I was in the living room with Vickie trying to help with the after Christmas stuff, and all of a sudden I got very hot, weak and sick. Guy & Clint came in and made me lie on the floor and put my head and feet up. It made a big difference and I felt better after a little bit. Then went to bed. Had to take nausea pill. Slept pretty good, restless on and off.

January 7th: Not too good yet. Laid around in bed till about 10:00 AM or so. Felt like eating and had small bowl of cereal. Still not feeling good, laid around some more. Went to Subway with Guy to get a sandwich. Felt a little better after I ate that, but I think the Subway sandwich was not a good thing to do. I was so hungry and ate it way to fast and of course it didn't digest well. Also, I had a half of piece of garlic bread tonight, not a good idea either.

January 8th: Boy was I right. Had a terrible night. Didn't sleep and ended up throwing up. Had heart burn all night. Stayed in bed most of morning. Got up and took a shower and got dressed. Still not feeling well but managed to take a ride with Guy to do some errands. Heartburn was not going away so called the doctor. She said I had to go to ER or see Dr. Kovats right away. Called Dr. Kovats office and they took me in, thank goodness. Did not want to go to ER. He gave me some stuff for gas and indigestion and told me I had to eat a little bit every two hours. The full meals were causing me the problems. I was not digesting quick enough. All has to do with chemo of course. I don't want to do this anymore!!"

Chemo Brain

Florence and I were walking out to the car after a short visit to a local Mall. Knowing that I left my car keys at home, I asked for hers. She stopped and started to rummage through her purse looking for the keys. I said, "What's wrong?"

Frustrated she answered, "I can't find my keys."

"Maybe they're in your pocket," I said.

"No, I always leave my keys in my purse." She paused for a moment and placed her hand in her pocket. Even more frustrated, she pulled the keys out and said, "I have Chemo Brain."

"Chemo brain? What's chemo brain?" "I don't know. I heard that at the treatment center. It has something to do with memory problems caused by taking chemotherapy."

Hmm! Chemo brain I thought to myself, another side effect? We got home, and the first thing I did was to Google "chemo brain."

Many people taking chemotherapy for cancer treatment have complained that they sometimes were in a fog, not able to concentrate, losing the ability to remember certain things. They believed the reason was related to the chemotherapy they were taking. What they were experiencing was what researchers call mild cognitive impairment. [49]The cause of mild cognitive impairment during cancer treatment isn't understood and doctors aren't sure what they can do about it.

Another term used by cancer patients was "chemo fog." Both terms, chemo brain and chemo fog, imply there is a relationship with cancer and chemotherapy. Women with breast cancer taking chemotherapy were the first to complain to their doctors about this. Still no one really knows if it's due to the chemo drugs they were taking. There are other factors such as stress and hormonal fluctuations, which could also be related.

To this day I never believed Florence suffered from chemo brain. However, research does show there is a noticeable number of cancer patients who do have memory issues. The memory changes are often subtle. Researchers find that people who report having memory difficulties tend to score in the normal ranges on tests of their cognitive ability. That makes it more difficult to understand, diagnose, and treat the memory changes.

[50]About twenty percent to thirty percent of people undergoing chemotherapy will experience cognitive impairment, although some studies report that at least half the participants had memory problems. One study found 35 percent of women with breast cancer had memory problems before beginning chemotherapy. Indeed, it's a perplexing problem. And, it isn't [50]clear which chemotherapy drugs are more likely to cause memory changes or if higher doses pose a bigger risk than do smaller ones. [50]It also isn't possible to predict who's more likely to have cognitive impairment after chemotherapy.

A number of factors can cause [50]temporary memory problems in people undergoing chemotherapy — making it difficult to identify the so-called "chemo brain" from the regular stresses of treatment. Temporary memory problems can, for the most part, be treated.

Some of the possible causes may include:

Low blood counts. If your blood counts are low, you may feel tired, making it difficult to concentrate.

Stress. Being diagnosed with cancer and starting treatment is stressful. Stress also makes concentrating difficult.

Medication - treat side effects. [50]Certain medications for treating side effects, including nausea and vomiting may cause drowsiness. When you're tired, it may take longer to complete tasks.

Lingering depression. [51]Depression is common in people with cancer. If your depression continues after your treatment, you might find it difficult to pay attention.

Lingering fatigue. [51]Fatigue is a side effect of several types of cancer treatment, including chemotherapy. Your fatigue might end when your cancer treatment ends although it can also continue after treatment.

Hormonal changes. Many cancer treatments may alter the normal hormonal balance in your body, causing cognitive changes. Hormonal changes are a side effect of some treatments and, with other treatments, are the intended way to treat your cancer.

Pain medications. Some pain medications cause drowsiness and difficulty concentrating. For most people, these side effects diminish or disappear once a proper dose of pain medication is established.

What really causes the memory changes?

Doctors don't know what causes the [52]cognitive changes associated with chemotherapy. It was previously thought that chemotherapy drugs didn't enter your brain, but were kept out by the blood-brain barrier, which separates chemicals that should be in your brain from those that shouldn't. But some researchers now suspect some chemotherapy drugs may be able to slip past the blood-brain barrier. This could potentially affect your brain and your memory.

What are chemo brain symptoms?

Word finding. Having problems reaching for the right word in conversation.

Memory. Short-term memory lapses such as not remembering where you put your keys or what you were supposed to buy at the store.

Multitasking. Example: talking with your grandkids and making dinner at the same time. [52]Chemotherapy may affect how well you're able to perform multiple tasks at once.

Learning. It might take longer to learn new things. Reading paragraphs over and over before you get the meaning.

Processing speed. Doing a task that once was quick and easy becomes slow and requires more effort.

So what about Florence and where is Florence in all of this?

The problem isn't that Florence can't remember where she put my keys; it's that once she finds the keys she still can't recall that she put them in her pocket. The concern is there a pattern of forgetfulness of significant events or responsibilities? The answer is no. Florence did finally remember she had placed the keys in her pocket, and there are no signs of cognitive impairment. She does not have chemo brain.

Could it be Alzheimer's setting in? There are several reasons for lapses of memory besides Alzheimer's. I bring up Alzheimer because Florence's mom suffered from this disease, and she, her siblings, and her dad know very well what her mom went through. Florence sometimes worries that Alzheimer's will strike, perhaps one of us, perhaps another member of her family. I regularly remind her when she notices that she is forgetting things more frequently, double check what is going on in your life. Stress and depression can cause memory problems, and it is common, not just among seniors. The loss of a friend or relative, and other major life changes, like breast cancer may also be a reason. "Honey," I would say to her, "There is a significant difference between forgetting where your keys to the car are and forgetting what your car looks like. Forgetting where you put your eyeglasses and forgetting that you have eyeglasses."

Florence was a little upset with the lost key episode, thinking she may have chemo brain. In an attempt to comfort her, I told her a "forgetful" story I had read somewhere. I said to her, "Two [53]elderly ladies had been friends for many decades. Over the years, they had shared all kinds of activities and adventures. Lately, their activities had been limited to meeting a few times a week to play cards. One day, they were playing cards when one looked at the other and said, "Now don't get mad at me. I know we've been friends for a long time, but I just can't think of your name! I've thought and thought, but I can't remember it. Please tell me what your name is." Her friend glared at her. [53]For at least three minutes. She just stared at her. Finally she said, "How soon do you need to know?"

Florence smiled at me and said, "I bet you'll forget that you told me this joke tomorrow." I did! So, the both of us have chemo brains! So what? One of us is taking chemotherapy, and the other is not. So what's up with that? The fact is Florence is fine and has the same mental lapses as all of us.

In Florence's Own Words

"Getting a little anxious about tomorrow, but excited to be getting the last Chemo done. I'm more prepared this time than the last, so hopefully with a positive attitude and knowing it's the last one will make it a little easier. Eating and drinking seem to make a big difference, so I plan to drink a lot more, if I can, and eat soft foods. This seems to be the worst I've felt, and for so long, during any of chemo sessions I've had, but I did make it through. Think positive think positive. I need to keep saying those words that Guy's high school coach "Stitch Vari" sent to me. "PMA - Positive Mental Attitude." I'm working really hard on that."

January 24th - The Sixth and Last Treatment Cycle

The sixth treatment, and the last! Wow, what a journey! Starting with her Mammogram on July 3rd, and now here we are, January 24th the end of her chemotherapy treatments. The morning started like all the previous mornings when we traveled to the treatment center. However, this time it was a little different. There were cautious optimism and some apprehension as we drove that familiar route. We talked very little, mostly about what we had planned for the remainder of the day. Somehow I knew she was thinking, even though this would be her last treatment, would it be as bad as the previous one?

We walked into the center and did what we always did. We said, "hello" to the receptionist, who will give Florence a big and loving hug as she has done so many times before. I usually am not a recipient of these hugs, but something tells me I will get one this morning. We signed the appointment calendar indicating Florence was here, and then sat down waiting to be called. We watch for a few minutes as the patients, one by one, are called into the treatment room.

It didn't take long until Florence was called. I followed her into the room where she sat in one of the chemo chairs. The nurse prepped her, took some blood for analysis, and then placed the chemo bags onto the pole directly behind her. Locating her access port, the nurse penetrated the skin with a small needle. She felt a little pinch. A tee was connected to the drip tube. Now it would start, a three-and-a-half hour infusion of the chemo drugs assigned to her protocol. I watched as I did so many times; I could not help but remember the first treatment back on October 4th. The tears, the stress, the apprehension, was this the best thing to do? It was indeed a very sad time for her - and me. Now, after all the treatments, here we are today with only three hours left to finish her chemotherapy, a part of her journey she can't wait to complete. She grasps that, for the next seven days or so, she will have to deal with the side effects, but she also knows, God willing, she will not have to deal with it again.

I left the treatment room and despite some tension sat in the waiting room, but also believing she would do well. I could not help but think this was to be a good day.

In Florence's Own Words

"I'm sitting here getting my treatment (three & half hours of drippings) and I'm thinking this is the last of the Chemo YEAA!! It hasn't been the most fun or the easiest, but there really has been a lot of humor in it - if you look at the positive side - and it's a good thing to do right now since I don't know what tomorrow or the next several days will bring, and I may be having some impure thoughts then.

The first bit of humor I remember was going bald. I look at my head everyday and unfortunately I'm not one of those "wow - you really are pretty bald" people. Then I look at the rest of my face and its quite swollen and bloated, and half of my eyelashes are gone (it was quite funny when I tried putting mascara on, it just didn't work with a few lashes, on the top left and a few lashes on the bottom right), my skin isn't quite the same and I get an extra big rash on it after Chemo. But the ultimate was, I got up a few days ago and the first thing I saw in the mirror was a big, very bright red flashing pimple (kind of Rudolph like) on the end of my nose. I started thinking, okay God, I guess I needed just a little more of a test. Not sure why, but okay. So then I started looking at the rest of this body. I look at my fingernails and I see red blotches under them. That looks bad enough, but 3 nails are starting to lift, so I may lose them, I'm praying they'll change their mind and stay. If I do lose them, I'm thinking some of those glittered gloves that Michael Jackson wears might be in order. I can't tell what's happening with my toenails. I've been keeping them polished so I can't see them. They hurt like my fingernails do, but what's a little pain here and there - ha! After checking myself from head to toe, I just started laughing out loud - maybe it was actually hysteria, I'm not quite sure.

The next funny thing was when I heard I would probably be going through the symptoms of menopause again. That was so funny to hear I think I just went into a trance. This was a real lift %&#*!!! You should have seen the look on Guy's face – deer in highlights?

I'm also reminded of the day I started to pass out (never passed out before in my life). Guy grabbed my shoulders and Clint grabbed my feet. They decided to get me to the bedroom after calling 911. All was good until they tried to get me though the bedroom door and decided to fold me up in half. That was a great idea for them but I couldn't breath and I couldn't get any air out to let them know I couldn't breath. Anyway, next thing I knew there were eight to ten paramedics around and in bed with me connecting monitors, checking my vitals, it was unbelievable.

After paramedics left, Josh came in and sat on the bed with me and started talking about Jessica's soccer game. In the middle of the conversation, he stopped and with a very serious face said; "Grandma, Jessica has major raging hormones" then shook his head and went back to the soccer story. I did everything to keep from bursting out laughing, which probably was not a great idea since it caused me major discomfort in my chest.

I'm just now realizing I could go on and on with lots more humorous times. I think it's the steroids that I take the day before, day of, and day after Chemo that has me wound up here. It makes me very high and happy for a while. I think I'm on the high and happy side right now. But the high and happy isn't all it's cracked up to be. I don't know how people take this voluntarily. The side effects are, you get quite antsy and have to keep moving around till you feel tired and when you try to sleep, and your legs won't stop jumping, you go back to clean the bathroom for the 6th time and start realizing the wax on the cabinets has gotten very thick looking, so you have to start taking the wax off. What is the fun part for these people? I keep looking but haven't found it yet. Anyway, I still have the Herceptin and radiation to go through, but I think that will be a breeze to get through - I hope."

It's Over!

Florence came through the doors with a smile on her face. I stood, and we both stared at each other. I immediately raised my right hand and gave her the "OK" sign, indicating it was over. No more, done, finished. I gave her a big emotional hug. The receptionist seeing this walked over and without hesitation gave a second congratulatory hug.

In Florence's Own Words

"Thursday January 24th: Got up this morning and didn't feel too good. My face was very swollen and very red. Was scared that Chemo might be cancelled because of this, but after talking to Dr. Shroff, I was good to go. Thank God. Everything went well and time went pretty quickly as I worked on an email to everybody almost the whole time I was there. I got a beautiful bouquet, twenty-four white roses, delivered to me back in the treatment room from my wonderful, wonderful husband. I love him soooooooo much. When I walked out the front door to leave, after treatment was done, I got quite a surprise. Guy & Janet and Clint & Vickie were waiting outside with balloons, chocolates, roses, a bottle of wine for Guy (wish I could have some), and a big poster that the kids made for me, and they were all blowing bubbles. I could not believe it. They all left work in the middle of the day to be there for me - wow. Being the very strong person that I'm not, of course I started crying. That day will be something I will never forget. The grandkids were still in school, so they couldn't be there. We celebrated with them at dinner that night). Even the receptionist came out and gave me a big hug. When I got home there was a beautiful bouquet of flowers from Theresa and Frank and Bev and Ken saying congratulations on ending my Chemo treatments. That was so neat!!! Unbelievable!!! Oh my, here come some more tears. Anyway, it was all more than wonderful. Again, what can I say about my family. I heard from my other brothers and their wives congratulating me on getting through these chemo treatments. Our son's, their wives (I call them my daughters, not daughters-in-law), and the grandkids, I can't even come up with the words for what they have done for both Guy and me. So much love!!!"

We both walked through the exit door and out to the parking lot and were surprised by our sons and their wives. What a treat for Florence and me. Our son Clint is spraying bubbles everywhere; one of them is waving a large poster signed by the grandkids and their parents, and; finally each of them gives Florence a hug. Yes, tears were flowing. It doesn't get any better than this. Oh, by the way, I finally got my hug from the receptionist.

After leaving the kids, we visited St. Margaret Mary's Church in Winter Park, fulfilling a promise we made to each other to say a prayer and give thanks for bringing Florence this far - safely. And to give thanks to all of our friends and family for their support and prayers these last six months. Florence's journey continues, and so far the journey has been and continues to be a remarkable and life changing event.

After her last treatment Florence, dealt with the side effects with a wonderful spirit. Her final chemo treatment was a concern to us since chemo treatment side effects previously have been tough for her. As it turned out, Florence did very well. The side effects were minimal, better than we expected. Actually, it seemed unbelievable how well she did.

Florence will continue taking Herceptin treatments, but instead of once every week, it will be once every three weeks. We learned she could tolerate a triple dose of Herceptin every three weeks rather than taking a single dose every week. If all goes well, she will complete the Herceptin treatments at the end of September.

In Florence's Own Words

"January 27th – 30th: Stayed in bed till about 3:00 PM today. Then went back to bed fairly early. Monday and Tuesday I lay around most of the day. Went to store with Guy for a little while, but that was all. Took a sleeping pill and slept well all night. Wednesday felt pretty good and stayed up all day (yea). Did some errands with Guy, nothing great today, but very tired still.

January 31st: Herceptin Treatment. Thursday - Had my first three doses at once. So far so good! Don't have to go back for three weeks now. That is so great.

February 1st - 12th: First 3 days felt okay, just a little under the weather. After that I've been feeling great. On the 10th we went to Carrabba's for dinner for Guy & Janet's anniversary and Vickie's birthday. I split the ravioli cheese pasta with Amanda and it was great. I had a little heartburn and took a GasX and it was gone. Enjoyed that meal so much, it's the first red sauce I've had since I found out I had breast cancer. I was so excited.

February 28th: Had my three doses of Herceptin today. Swelled up a little and got red rash on face, but that's all. Not bad at all. Started with a cold today and was afraid I wouldn't be able to get treatment, but they said I could. That was a relief.

I had my consultation today at Dr. Diamond's Office for radiation treatments. Met with Dr. Diamond's Assistant and she explained everything to Guy and me about what to expect with the treatments. She felt a lump when she checked the breast area and it scared me at first when she told me she felt it. But she said it was nothing to worry about, that it was probably just scar tissue from my surgery. I'll be seeing Dr. Weise, my surgeon, this Tuesday March 4th. He will be able to tell me more."

Radiation Treatment - The Journey Continues

Florence met with the Radiation Oncologist, Dr. Diamond, to start planning radiation treatments. Radiation treatment is called Local Treatment and is aimed at the original site of her tumor. The thinking is, there could have been bad guys (cancer cells) floating around after the surgical procedure was completed. This again, is a precautionary treatment, and if they are indeed there they will be eradicated (goodbye to the bad guys) by the radiation.

After a physical exam and a review of her medical records, the first requirement was to pin point the area of treatment. This was done today (Friday) and involved the following:

First, a CT scan was taken of her chest to define the treatment area. To ensure the radiation beam is aimed correctly, a special mold (cast) of parts of her body was created. The size of a pillow, the mold is designed to keep her still by holding her head and her left arm in the exact location during the radiation treatment. Florence was nervous and a little anxious during this process, but I told her I would keep the mold for her so she could use it during her nap times at home. I'm sure I didn't score any points with that one because her response included some explicit words. To be a comic you need to learn about timing. Timing is everything! Again, so much to learn!

Next Friday, March 7, Florence will make another visit to the Radiation Center where the Radiation Therapist will mark the treatment area with freckle-sized dots of ink on her left breast. The dots will remain there forever. Based on the simulation and other test Dr. Diamond will decide how much radiation will be needed.

This state-of-art technology was developed to provide a more accurate way of giving external radiation, and to allow the doctors to focus the radiation on the site where the tumor was originally removed. The technology is called IMRT for Intensity Modulated Radiation Therapy. IMRT allows the strength of the beams to be changed to lessen damage to normal body tissues, resulting in fewer side effects. Remember all of this, as it will be a question on the quiz I will be sending all of you later – just kidding...

In Florence's Own Words

"February 29th: I went back to Dr. Diamond's office today for what they call "the simulation". It includes getting a cat scan and marking the breast area for radiation. They molded a thing (kind of like a very solid/hard pillow) around my neck, shoulders and top of arms. It's made just for the person getting radiation, so it will be mine only, everyday I go. I go back next Friday, March 7th and have a dye injected into the marked areas, which are five. The dye leaves what they call a tattoo about the size of a freckle in each of the marked spots so they can target those spots every time during treatment. I have little wire's there now. Then I start the radiation treatments the following Monday, March 10th. Its pretty amazing what they do. When the nurse was examining my left breast, she found that lump I talked about earlier, close to surgery scar. She also thought it might be scar tissue. Have an appointment with Dr. Wiese on March 4th. He will be checking that out. The appointment was originally for follow-up after chemo was done.

March 4th Tuesday - Appointment with Dr. Wiese today. Dr. Wiese checked the lump on my left breast and said I'd need to have a mammogram and sonogram done. He wasn't quite sure what it was, and wanted to have it checked. Everything else was good. My port was still looking very good. We made appointments for mammogram and sonogram for tomorrow."

March 5th - Mammogram Tests . . .

Many [55]radiologists recommend that patients have a mammogram of the treated breast (especially if the lesion has calcifications; tiny calcium deposits) immediately before and six months after the completion of radiation treatments. Radiation therapy and chemotherapy both cause changes in the skin and breast tissues that show up on the mammogram and may make the mammogram results more difficult to interpret. These changes are required to be at their peak at six months after the radiation therapy is finished.

Today's mammogram test will be the first for Florence since the initial one that found the lesion in her left breast back in July. Future mammograms will be compared to this mammogram to follow the healing and to check for cancer recurrence. [56]As part of her continuing treatment she will expect to have a mammogram of the treated breast about six months after finishing her radiation treatment. This six-month mammogram will become the new "standard" against which future mammograms of the remaining breast tissue are compared. Six months later, she can expect to have her usual yearly mammogram of both breasts. From this point on, Dr. Shroff may say that yearly mammograms are sufficient. [56]Or, she may recommend that the treated breast still get a mammogram every six months for the next few years.

Women who have had breast cancer are more likely to develop a second breast cancer so it will be necessary for Florence to get these screening mammograms. [56]The screening mammograms on the other breast are especially critical, because having cancer in one breast raises your risk of developing cancer in the other.

As always it's never easy for me to accompany Florence to yet another test procedure. I find myself concerned and wondering if she will be in any pain. More than that, what will the outcome be for her?

Although there were concerns with all the previous tests and treatments, this visit seems to bother me more. Maybe it's because we're imaging the location where we found the original tumor back in early July. Would the results show a new one even though she has just finished 18 weeks of chemotherapy? Has the weekly dose of Herceptin been a complete waste? What if they do find new lesions? What do we do? Where do we go from here? I pray to myself,

"Oh God, keep me strong today, we're both in your hands. Keep me from thinking negative. Give me the positive mental attitude You have always given me and Florence."

We entered the Florida Radiology Imaging Center, checked in with the receptionist and sat down waiting for her turn to be called. It didn't take long until she was asked to come into the lab. I stood up to follow her, but the nurse technician said, "Sorry Mr. Carbonneau, you're not allowed to go with her." I started to give her all the reasons I should be with her, but I chose to be quiet and sit down and wait, - even though I really wanted to be with her. I placed my two fingers on my lips, raised them to her and whispered, "I love you." She immediately reciprocated, "I love you too," and proceeded through the doors.

In Florence's Own Words

"March 5th: Had mammogram and sonogram done this morning! The only thing they could tell me was, it was not a solid mass, but a liquid. That was good news as far as we knew. It could be cystic, but as far as we know its not cancer. Guy talked to Bob Baratta and he said it's not uncommon after surgery to have that. We have an appointment with Dr. Wiese on Wednesday the 12th for exact results and what will be done about it. He said to go on with appointments for radiation treatments. Both Guy and I didn't sleep very well last night. It was really scary not knowing exactly what that lump was, but we both feel a little relieved right now that it didn't sound like cancer. Boy, it's amazing what your mind can do when your waiting for results - not fun.

Friday March 7th: Follow-up at Dr. Diamond's office for marking/ tattooing breast area for treatments! It was a lot easier than I expected. The 5 needle injections were not bad at all. Two were a little sensitive, but nothing really to complain about. The technicians were really nice."

Waiting for Mammogram test results . . .

It didn't take long for her to complete the test and return back to the waiting room. I asked the nurse how long before we would have the results. She indicated that the radiologist would talk to us as soon as he was finished writing his findings. Approximately fifteen minutes went by when the radiologist came through the door and said the following to us: "Mrs. Carbonneau, the mammogram showed no new masses or suspicious areas in your left breast. We want to see you again in six months after you finish your radiation treatments."

After all the apprehensions, the anxieties, the news is good. The news is excellent! God continues to walk with us.

The actual Unilateral Diagnostic Mammogram findings are as follows:

"Indication: Palpable area in left lumpectomy site.

Findings: Ultrasound of the lumpectomy site reveals stroma/ hematoma fluid collection measuring 2.8 x 3.1 x 1.3 cm. This is quite superficial and is palpable. This corresponds to the patient's palpable area. Six-month follow-up left-sided unilateral diagnostic mammogram is recommended or as soon as possible after patient receives radiation therapy and can tolerate it.

BIRADS Category 2: BENIGN FINDING

Good News!

Yes indeed! Again, God walks with the both of us.

Florence will continue to get the high-quality mammograms and have a clinical breast exam by her health care provider on a regular basis. This will be the most effective way to detect a recurrence in her breast.

I know many individuals have concerns about taking radiation treatments due to the risk of cancer; however, the risk is slight, and the benefit of an accurate diagnosis far outweighs the risk. Also, the effective radiation dose from a mammogram is about 0.7 mSv, which is about the same as the average person receives from background radiation in three months.

I sense the reader wants more information on radiation exposure, so here we go. Remember you can always skip this tech stuff if you want.

The [60]scientific unit of measurement for radiation dose, commonly referred to as effective dose, is the millisievert (mSv).

Because different tissues and organs have varying sensitivity to radiation exposure, the real dose to various parts of the body from an x-ray procedure varies. [62]The term effective dose is used when referring to the dose averaged over the entire body.

We are exposed to radiation from [61]natural sources all the time. The average person in the U.S. receives an effective dose of about 3 mSv per year from naturally occurring radioactive materials and cosmic radiation from outer space. These natural "background" doses vary throughout the country.

People living in the plateaus of Colorado or New Mexico receive about 1.5 mSv more per year than those living near sea level. The added dose from cosmic rays during a coast-to-coast round trip flight in a commercial airplane is about 0.03 mSv. [63]Altitude plays a significant role, but the largest source of background radiation comes from radon gas in our homes (about 2 mSv per year). Like other sources of background radiation, exposure to radon varies widely from one part of the country to another.

To [62]explain it in simple terms, we can compare the radiation exposure from one chest x-ray as equivalent to the amount of radiation exposure one experiences from our natural surroundings in 10 days.

The above information is provided by, "Radiology Info" (www. radiologyinfo.org), radiology information resource for patients.

First Radiation Treatment...

On Monday, March 10th Florence started her first radiation treatment. The treatment lasted approximately fifteen minutes. Florence will repeat the process daily; Monday thru Friday, for a period of six weeks. She should complete the treatments around April 21st. Florence expects to tolerate the radiation treatments with little discomfort, maybe some slight radiation burn, akin to sunburn. Fatigue will continue to be a factor.

In Florence's Own Words

"Monday March 10th: Radiation treatments start today. Had to wait a little as the radiation machine was cold and it took a little time for it to warm up. Then there was a problem with one of the leads and they had to get that corrected. When we finally started, it didn't take long at all. Most of the time was getting my body exactly into the right position. The pillow helps with that, and keeping the head and chest area from moving. The actual radiation time when all that is done is just five minutes or so. So the total time from laying down to getting up is not longer than 15 minutes. It was really easy, felt nothing.

Tuesday, March 11th: Today was very fast and easy. Everything was working, so didn't have to wait. Felt nothing.

Wednesday, March 12th: Radiation and then appointment with Dr. Wiese, regarding mammogram and sonogram results.

Dr. Wiese said the lump was liquid left over from surgery. Thank God! It will go away in time, but if it seems to get any worse to let him know."

Receiving radiation therapy is like going into a tanning booth.

Over the past decade, [64]engineers have learned how to shape high-energy x-rays from machines called linear accelerators, modulate the beams' intensity, and guide them straight to the patient's tumor with the aid of high-tech imaging systems. This results in better treatment outcomes, and a decrease in harmful side effects. I knew that - right!

Florence continues on this phase of her journey. Both of us find the days going by so fast it seems mind-boggling. She continues to do well with the radiation therapy and, with the exception of a slight burning sensation, she continues to be positive. She was told by the radiation technician her skin would be uncomfortably raw, and she would need to use a skin care product. Her mild pinkness, itching, and burning, was easily taken care of by applying an aloe preparation. She would spread the cream thinly over the affected area three times a day.

As each day goes by, it's one more day behind her on her way to completing this part of her journey. Thirty-four treatments! ETC - Expected Time of Completion, April 23rd.

Bad Hair Day

As you know, Florence, during chemo, started to have what she calls "bad hair days." Recently her hair has shown some activity, meaning it's starting to grow back. Florence has always tried to hide her hair loss from me, but last week, she called me. "Yo, Guy?" Never has she said to me - "Yo, Guy." "Yo, Guy," I thought to myself, where did that come from? I walked over to the bathroom door where Florence was staring at me with a big smile. She burst out laughing at the expression on my face. Florence's hair was indeed growing back. Each and every hair strand stood straight up one inch above her head. Do you remember pictures of monkeys? - Nope, I'm not going there. We could not stop laughing each time she stared in the mirror. I think it's one of those times when you had to be there.

In Florence's Own Words

"Monday March 17th: Met with Dr. Diamond, everything going well with radiation so far!

Thursday March 20th: Herceptin day. Had radiation at 8:30 AM and then went in for three doses of Herceptin. No problems except, about fifteen minutes before I was done I felt a little nauseated, but I think it was because I hadn't eaten. We stopped for a bagel on the way home and I felt much better."

Easter - Twenty-Three Radiation Treatments Left . . .

Easter celebration was wonderful with all our family. Again, the ten of us sit in the same pew at St. Stephen, celebrating Mass together. Florence and I continue to be blessed and thank God everyday for our family and friends.

Florence is handling the radiation treatments well; the only complaint has been fatigue. Florence's doctors tell us the fatigue is caused by the previous chemotherapy treatments, the residuals of which will hang around for some time. As I mentioned previously in this book, chemotherapy kills fast dividing cancer cells. [65]The problem is it also kills some fast dividing healthy cells in the body, [66] like some cells in the bone marrow that maintain the supply of white cells in the blood. As the [65]bone marrow cells recover from the effects of chemotherapy, the white blood count (WBC) starts rising again. That's a good thing. White blood cells are responsible for protecting the body from infections. When WBC counts are low, there is an increased risk of infections and other issues. Rest will be necessary as the body is healing. Especially when the body is telling Florence she needs the rest.

March 24th - MUGA Scan

Florence has been on Herceptin since last October. Her final treatment will end in late September. One of the toxic side effects of Herceptin is it may cause heart issues. Prior to starting Florence's chemotherapy and Herceptin treatment, Dr. Shroff had ordered a MUGA test to establish a base on her heart functions. After six months of Herceptin treatments, it was time for a second MUGA test to evaluate the condition of her heart. Would there be any issues after taking Herceptin for the last six months? Hopefully not! It took a few days to receive the results, causing anxieties for the both of us. In the past, waiting for results for any of Florence's test has always been difficult. Finally, the news . . . it was good. Florence's heart had tolerated the treatments, and it was safe for her to continue the Herceptin treatments. Six more months to go and Florence will be through with all the chemotherapeutic treatments. At the end of September, we will have to find a way to celebrate the end of Florence's journey.

Wednesday April 23rd -
The Last Radiation Treatment

There have been many wonderful moments in Florence's journey, and the following is one of them. On April 23, Florence finished her last radiation treatment. She said to me on that wonderful and optimistic day, "Another one of those happiest days of my life. I even received a diploma from the radiation nurses and technicians for completing my treatments. WOW! It was like graduating from high school."

Florence was very good about watching out for side effects during the treatments. I, too, was somewhat concerned even though the research indicated most patients tolerated the treatments. As expected, Florence did experience redness and tenderness around the treatment area. It didn't start until after a couple weeks, and she knew immediately what to do. She consulted with the radiation oncologist who recommended an Aloe gel, a hypoallergenic gel that has no known side effects. Aloe gel helps with radiation burns. When applied on the affected area of the skin, it creates a protective coating, which speeds up the healing process and relieves pain. The best news she said, "This also will pass and September is just around the corner."

CA27.29 - Tumor Marker

During the course of treatments, Florence had blood drawn to test her red blood count (RBC) and the white blood count (WBC). The principal purpose of WBCs is to fight disease. Increased levels are often an indication that the body is fighting infection. It is common for levels to decrease during chemotherapy.

Another test performed was called [67]CA27.29. CA27.29 is a tumor marker test similar to the CA15-3 that is found in the blood of most breast cancer patients. CA27.29 levels may be used in conjunction with other procedures, such as mammograms to check for recurrence in women previously treated for stage II and stage III breast cancer. Tumor markers are substances released by cancer cells created by the body in response to cancer cells. This test is used to evaluate how well Florence has responded to her treatment and to check for the possibility of recurrence.

There is, however, disagreement about the ability of CA27.29 to detect recurrence after curative treatments. One trial in patients at high risk for recurrence of breast cancer (stage II or III) found that CA27.29 was highly specific and sensitive in detecting preclinical metastasis. The average time from initial elevation of CA27.29 to onset of symptoms was five months. Dr. Shroff, however would like as much information as possible, at her disposal, if signs of recurrence should manifest itself. If Florence's CA27.29 level was to elevate, it may lead to the imaging of probable sites of metastasis, and then decisions about treatment will need to take into account other factors, not strictly a rising CA27.29 level. A standard CA27.29 level is usually less than 38 to 40 U/ml (units/milliliter), depending on where the lab-test is done because anything under 40 is considered typical. Florence had five CA27.29 tests during her treatments. The CA27.29 level never exceeded 13.

In Florence's Own Words

"Note: I met several people during this time (besides friends and family) who were so nice and very caring. But there were three so far who I felt made a difference for me. The first one was a girl named Lesley Harris who Guy first

met at St. Steven's at a Wednesday morning mass (he goes to mass everyday since I got my diagnoses). She tapped him on the back one morning at mass and said she thought he looked like he had a lot on his mind. After church they talked and he found out she had had lung cancer and one lung was removed. She was in remission. Then he told her about me. The following Wednesday she spoke with Guy again (she only goes to mass on Wednesdays during the week) only this time she had a blanket that she made and asked Guy to give it to me. The following Wednesday she gave him another present for me, another blanket, along with several little things in a pretty bag. Again, after Guy was at mass, Fr. George called him over and said "Lesley asked me to give you this". It was another gift bag with a little angel, a block-buster gift card for $30 (she told Guy to go get some fun movies for us to watch) and little note cards, along with a note her daughter had written to her when she found out she had cancer. Then believe it or not, on another Wednesday she sent a gift bag home with Guy and this time it had 2 huge bottles of shampoo and scalp treatment (which she said she thinks helped a lot when her hair started coming back), nail hardener, and several other little things for me. During all of this, I finally got to meet her one morning at Barney's for coffee. We hugged when we met, and we just clicked/bonded. We talked about this closeness we both felt several times when we met again. Was it the cancer? Not sure, but that bonding stayed with us till the very end. She is wonderful. She's only about forty-two and has two daughters about eight and ten years old. She recently found out that she has some spots on her other lung and went to Boston to see another specialty doctor. When she came back she said he was great and they would be doing some more tests on her. After the test, she and her husband and her girls decided to take a week and go see her brother and sister-in-law in Colorado. She was so excited. She is very close to her brother and says he has been amazing with her during all of this. She is supposed to call us when she gets back to get together for lunch or something. I bought her a Lenox angel that said, "When I count my blessings, I count two for you" and a pretty candle. She truly has been an angel for both Guy and me.

The second person is the lady (about my age) receptionist at the Chemo Center. From the first day I started Chemo she has come out and hugged me. I think she noticed how nervous I was, but continues to do this every time I go there (I will be seeing her every three weeks for Herceptin through September). I haven't seen her do it with anyone else. She has even come over and sat with Guy and me a couple of times. She was so excited when I finished my Chemo treatments. She even came outside when the kids surprised me that day with flowers, balloons, etc. She is getting married April 19th and is very excited about it. I bought her a really pretty blue (Boca Kasta) candleholder and of course candles. I hope she likes it. I just wanted to thank her for what she had done for me.

The third lady (probably in her early fifties) is a lady I met when I started my radiation treatments. Her name is Judy. She was an Attorney in Mississippi for years and then moved to Florida to be with her daughter. She now works for The American Society of Education. She was such a lift and we had some fun conversations during this time. Probably will never see her again, but when she finished her last treatment she was so very excited. I gave her a little angel and wished her the best of luck with her future.

I have to add here my friend Carolyn. From the first day she heard I had breast cancer, she called me at least once a week. She also had breast cancer about a year and a half before I was diagnosed. She is such a lift every time she calls. She is very humorous and at the same time very compassionate. She has no idea how much these calls mean to me.

April 14th Monday: Happy Birthday Mom! Went for radiation treatments. Met with Dr. Diamond and everything was still going good. I started to get some redness (like sunburn) this past week and now I have little bumps on the red area. I've been using aloe on it everyday and it seems to be working, just a little in that breast area.

Today I also went to a "look good, feel good" event at the radiation center. It was really fun. There were only three other women there. We got a bag full of make-up and there was a guy (named Gary) who showed us how to use it. He was a riot and said he was gay. He did a great job. I must have gotten about $250 or $300 items of make-up for free. It was worth going to. Gary also cut hair, so he trimmed my wig for me. It looks much better. Anyway, it was a lot of fun.

April 15th: Had radiation and they did some extra prep for more targeted area. So, they drew on me again. The good news is this means I'm very close to the end of this, just seven more days to go. YEA!!!

April 22nd: Hip-hip-hooray!!! Had final radiation today. The last five days were in a different radiation room. This radiation is called "boosters". It is aimed at the scar area only and is very quick. Maybe five minutes. Everything went very well through all of the radiation. I did get the "sunburn" and it was a little uncomfortable at times, but other than that nothing but a little tired towards the end of the treatments (fifth and sixth week). All of the staff, especially Susie, Sarah, Chris, Al, and Stacie, was absolutely great. They are the kind of people needed in these areas. I never saw one of them without a smile and something nice to say everyday. They gave me a certificate congratulating me on my treatments. It was really cute. I bought them a big box of donuts to thank them and they enjoyed that.

Clint & Vickie had Guy & Janet and the kids come over for a celebration dinner tonight. It was stuffed shells stuffed with spinach and mozzarella cheese. It was great. The kids made me a really cute card. It was a cat without hair and then a cat with lots of wild funny hair. It apparently reminded them of me. It was funny. They are so great, such good grandkids, I really love them."

May 9th - Florence Starts Hormonal Treatments

Dr. Shroff started Florence on an additional treatment program. She will take Arimidex, a drug in pill form, each day for the next five years that will further reduce the chances of a cancer recurrence. Remember, this past year, all the drugs, all the radiation and all the side effects that were inherent with the treatments, had been designed to remove chances of a recurrence.

Arimidex therapy prevents natural estrogen from reaching cancer cells that may be around. The bad guys (cancer cells) depend on estrogen to grow. By reducing the amount of estrogen, there is less available to stimulate tumor growth - that is a good thing.

In Florence's Own Words

"May 9th: Started taking Arimidex today and will continue daily for five years. Yikes!!! Things are still good right now."

Arimidex is called an Aromatase Inhibitors (AI). Hormones in Florence's body called androgens are changed into estrogen by an enzyme called Aromatase. The aromatase enzyme is involved in the production of the female sex hormone, Oestrogen. In women who have passed menopause Oestrogen is mainly produced by aromatase. In [69]postmenopausal women, the aromatase enzyme converts the sex hormones androstenedione (produced by the ovary), and testosterone, into Oestrogen. What Arimidex does cleverly is to prevent this conversion by blocking the action of the aromatase enzyme. This causes Oestrogen levels in the body to fall.

Many breast cancers are sensitive to Oestrogen, and they [69] need this hormone to grow. These types of breast cancers are termed hormone receptor positive. Florence's cancer was hormone receptor positive. [69]Oestrogen binds to Oestrogen receptors on the breast cancer cells and causes changes within the cells that result in faster growth of the cancer.

By lowering the levels of Oestrogen in the body, Arimidex effectively [69]starves the breast cancer cells, thus helping to stop them from growing. Preventing breast cancer from spreading to other areas of the body will reduce the risk of developing cancer in the other breast.

Arimidex Side Effects

Arimidex has been studied thoroughly in clinical trials, in which a group of people taking the medication has had side effects documented. As with any medicine, side effects are possible, however, not everyone who takes the medication, [68]Arimidex, experiences side effects. In fact, most people tolerate it quite well. If side effects do occur, in most cases, they are minor and either require no treatment or can be easily treated by your healthcare provider.

Florence will start her Arimidex treatment May 9th and finish sometime in May of 2013. At that time, with God's help, she will be five plus years cancer free.

May 31st - A Very Special Day

"Happy Birthday, Florence." With that said, the waiter gave Florence a box decorated with a ribbon and a birthday card that said,

"What lies behind us and what lies before us are tiny matters compared to what lies within us."
- Emerson.
I love you, Guy

After Florence finished her radiation treatments, I planned a way that would celebrate not only her birthday, but also how far she had come in the last twenty-two months. Her birthday was just around the corner, and what better way than to surprise her with a trip to a restaurant that has always been very special to the both of us, "The Old Angler's Inn" in Potomac, Maryland. For this surprise to work I would need an excuse to visit Washington, DC, and attend a meeting with a client. Florence, in most cases, had traveled with me on business trips, so this trip to her, was just another trip that she and I would enjoy together. The meeting went well on Friday, and on Saturday, the day of her birthday, we enjoyed sightseeing at nearby Middleburg, Virginia. That evening I asked her to dress up and get ready for an enjoyable evening. "Where are you taking me?" she said, with a very contagious smile.

"Never mind, you'll know when you get there."

"What about my hair, or lack of?"

"Honey," I said, "Pick the hair of your choice." Oops! I can't believe I just said that . . .

"What I meant to say is you're so good at getting dressed up, I'm sure you'll do what's right for your head." Oops, again.

What is wrong with me? She had brought a few wigs with her, each of which looks great on her. I looked at her to see if I had offended her, but being the classy lady that she is, she turned and said,

"OK, I'll be a blonde tonight. Or maybe, I'll be a brunette."

She was kidding with me and knew I was uncomfortable with what I had said. Even though she was practically bald, she had come to accept it and found excellent ways to make her head look great with the wigs she had. We both laughed together, and that became the start of a wonderful evening.

During our drive to the restaurant, Florence started to recognize the surroundings. She looked at me with a huge smile but didn't say anything. As we approached the driveway Florence saw the sign, "Welcome to Old Angler's Inn." We were escorted to a table underneath a lovely oak next to a small pond. She looked at me and said one word, "Wow!"

You could not ask for a better evening, a full moon, the flowers in and around the pond were in bloom, and in different colors. It indeed was a beautiful evening, but again anything God creates is always perfect. I looked at her and said one word, "Wow!"

A short time later, as we both were enjoying a martini, a waiter approached the table and said, "Happy Birthday, Florence," and gave her a decorated box along with a card. "Now you know the rest of the story."

In Florence's Own Words

May 31st: Today is my birthday. We are in Reston, VA right now leaving for Orlando tomorrow, Amanda's birthday. Have to mention here. Every year Amanda calls me a few days before my birthday and says: "Grandma, where should we go to celebrate our birthday?" Her birthday is the first of June. She is thirteen (I think), right now and she still calls and asks that question. I can't believe at this age she still wants to celebrate together. How lucky am I? And we will be home tomorrow to celebrate together.

Guy had meetings in Reston, Virginia and Westchester County, NY this past week. After Westchester, we headed back to Reston. Guy surprised me and took me to "The Olde Angler's Inn" for dinner. This was a favorite place for him and I when we lived in Reston many years ago. It was wonderful! Such a beautiful night! It was a little cool, but we sat outside. He had the waiter bring me a gift, which was a male and female angel and it says Love on it. I love it. It was a very special birthday. I can't believe how much Guy loves me, and I love him.

Several days after we got home, we met Lesley Harris (whom we've become very attached to) for coffee at a local coffee house. She handed me a birthday card. I asked how she knew it was my birthday, and she said: "a little birdie told me". Guy said he doesn't remember saying anything about my birthday to her, but maybe he did. Anyway, after reading the card, there was a little note saying that we had two tickets to see "Mama Mia" on August

16th. I couldn't believe it. I did everything to keep from crying. I didn't know how to thank her. When I went home and told the kids, I just started crying. It really hit me what an amazing person Lesley is. I've wanted to see that play ever since it came out. I worry about Lesley. She is going for another doctor's visit in Boston the week of June 16th. I can't wait till she gets back to hear how it all went. She's pretty private with all of this. She tells us some, but we're sure not all. She always says "I feel great and I'm doing fine", then changes the subject. She visits Father George and talks to him a lot. She really likes him, and I think she tells him all. We pray for her all the time."

Intimacy!

At the start of Florence's journey, I learned quickly to give her my undivided attention and to listen to her. Often I have taken the time to talk to her. Sometimes it's to tell her what's happening with her. Sometimes it's to check up on how she's doing, and sometimes it's just to say, "I'm here for you. I love you." Florence needed me to acknowledge her feelings; she needed to know that I understood what she was saying. Listening wasn't my best attribute, but I would learn. I learned also to be thoughtful about the small things, not always successfully, but I tried. So many times I stopped and took a good look at what she was doing in her world. But, I did more than notice. I tried very hard to participate.

There was a lot going on at first: the diagnosis, surgery decision, and all the medical protocols. I learned quickly to understand her emotions. When she was upset or frustrated, I realized that these emotions were her way of letting me know she needed me. There was a need so many times to be close to her and to touch her, a nonsexual touch that would communicate a genuine caring, and that I loved her more than just her body. But how do you maintain a sense of intimacy in a relationship when your wife is reeling from the detection of a potentially lethal condition? When her optimism and confidence is greatly tested? I wanted her to know I was here, and I would take care of her, but it was difficult. Sometimes she was frustrated and overwhelmed, about everything that was going on. I knew however, our intimacy had always been on the deepest level: when I let her get into my soul and I got into hers, we were together, and we would reveal who we are to each other. When we talk about everything and anything, and when we shared our opinions and perspectives, we really were together. This devotion was built with a strong sense of security and intimacy in our relationship.

In Florence's Own Words

"Thursday June 12th: Herceptin infusion today! Met with Dr. Shroff before treatment. I told her I have been getting a lot of uncomfortable pain on the right side of my hip (when I had a scan months ago, I was told I had

some arthritis there), which sometimes goes down the right side of my leg and across my ankle. I also told her I had some bone stiffness in my body. I was worried it was a side effect from the Arimidex. She thinks the bone stiffness is, but not the back or leg pain. She scheduled a Dexa Scan for Monday June 16th.

I met a girl who sat next to me during treatment today. Boy, I continue to realize how lucky I have been through all of these treatments. Nine years ago she was diagnosed with a very rare stomach cancer. In fact, she had to go to the Moffitt Cancer Center in Tampa, FL where they finally found a surgeon in this particular field. She was told she only had a twenty-five percent chance to live and it would be very difficult for her to go through her treatments. She immediately told the doctor she was going for a fifty percent chance to live and she wanted them to do whatever was necessary to get her started. She had her stomach removed and was in the hospital for quite a while after her surgery. When she was released she started her Chemotherapy at home for the next 5 months. It was twenty-four hours a day for that five months with only approximately a one minute stopping point after every twenty-four hours to clean her port and then start the next twenty-four hour treatment. She also had radiation at the same time. She had to be fed through tubes in her stomach area. She obviously was very, very sick during this time. She also had several hallucinations during these treatments. One specific one she recalled was; she called her then nine year old son into the room telling him to hurry up so he could see the ninja's jumping from tree to tree outside her window. Her son has just now turned nineteen. Well it has been nine years since this all started. She still goes once a month, since this all started, to get red blood cell shots, since her red blood level continues to stay low. Occasionally she has to get iron injections. That is what she was getting today. She is a very pretty lady, I'd say in her late forties and is Japanese.

She is very religious and credits that, and her husband and son, for getting her through these last nine years. She is very tiny and frail looking, but has a tough "I'm going to live" attitude. When she talked about her husband, he reminded me of Guy. He has been by her side since day one. We both talked about what an amazing impact they were for us and wondered how people with no support could get through something like this. We both felt so blessed and reconfirmed how lucky we are to have our husbands, our family, and our spirituality."

June 12, – Oncologist Appointment

Today is Florence's Herceptin treatment day. After today, she has five more treatments remaining, the last scheduled for September. One of the reasons for consulting with Dr. Shroff, her Oncologist, was Florence has been complaining of bone pain, mostly around her right shoulder and her feet. Other issues were discussed that included hot flashes and fatigue. Dr. Shroff concluded that most of the complaints were due to Arimidex, the pill she has been taking each day for the last thirteen months. Although Arimidex has been studied thoroughly in clinical trials, there have been some common side effects. About fifteen percent have bone pain, and twelve percent have joint pain. Between thirty six percent complain of hot flashes, and about nineteen percent complain of weakness or fatigue. Florence will continue to take Arimidex each day, for the next four years. Also, Dr. Shroff ordered a Dexa scan to measure bone density.

In Florence's Own Words

"Friday June 13th: Yesterday when I got home I didn't feel too great and was very tired. Today was not a good day for me. I had a very hard time getting up this morning and felt very tired and cranky all day. I tried to stay away from everybody.

Saturday June 14th: What a difference today is. Woke up at 7:30 AM and I'm feeling very well. It always seems to take a day or two after Herceptin to get back to myself. Tomorrow is Father's Day and I want to enjoy it with Guy and the kids and grandkids."

June 16th - DEXA Scan . . .

When Florence was first diagnosed, her oncologist focused on beating her malignancy. This was the priority and the most important task. Her treatment protocol included chemotherapy, and one of several concerns with cancer treatments is; it could have a negative effect by limiting or eliminating her hormones from circulating in her body. The hormone, estrogen, is an essential regulator of bone building cells. The lack of estrogen could cause bone deterioration or bone loss. So, one could say, it is a cancer side effect and needs to be dealt with. Dr. Shroff ordered the Dexa scan, a non-invasive test that requires very little preparation for Florence.

DEXA scans are the most commonly used test to measure bone density. It is one of the most accurate ways to diagnose Osteopenia or Osteoporosis. Florence's Dexa scan results indicated Osteopenia.

Osteopenia is a condition where bone mineral density is lower than normal. It is considered by many doctors to be a precursor to Osteoporosis. Like Osteoporosis, Osteopenia occurs more frequently in post-menopausal women as a result of the loss of estrogen. It can also be exacerbated by, not only her cancer treatments, but lifestyle factors such as lack of exercise, excess consumption of alcohol, smoking or some medications such as those prescribed for asthma.

However, not every person diagnosed with Osteopenia will develop Osteoporosis. Specifically, Osteopenia is defined as a bone mineral density T-Score between -1.0 and -2.5. Bone mineral density or BMD is a measure of the amount of minerals (mainly calcium) contained in a certain volume of bone. Calcium gives bones their strength and helps prevent fractures. A BMD test, also called a bone mass measurement, is used to measure bone density and can determine fracture risk for osteoporosis.

Florence's BMD T-Score was -1.8 on her left hip and -1.5 on her right hip. A T-score of -1.0 or higher is considered normal. A score of -1.0 and greater than -2.5 is defined as having Osteopenia. [72]A score of -2.5 or lower, meaning a bone density that is two-and-a-half standard deviations below the mean of a thirty year old woman is defined as having Osteoporosis.

In Florence's Own Words

"Monday June 16th: Had a Dexa Scan this morning to check bone density. This is done for three reasons. The first is from my complaint to Dr. Shroff on June 12th for bone pain and stiffness. The second is because sometimes after chemotherapy you can get bone loss in your body. The third is because Arimidex can also cause bone loss. I'll have to have this test done about every two years to make sure I'm not getting any bone loss. Test came back that I have Osteopenia. Its pre Osteoporosis and I probably had it for years. Nothing to worry about!

June 17th – 23rd: Started getting very, very tired again and very agitated. Got very, very depressed this week also. Not sure if this is the medicine or not, but need to keep track to see if this occurs again."

June 20th - Coffee with Lesley

It's been a while since we have last seen Lesley, and we were both looking forward to seeing her again. It was a beautiful morning; the sun was bright, the air was cool, a perfect morning to have coffee together at the local coffee house as we have previously done so often. As we entered the coffee house, Florence saw Lesley with a big smile on her face. It was one of those smiles that showed love and gratitude for the friendship they each had for each other. They both hugged each other as Florence said, "Hi Lesley." I stared at the both of them. Each had a tear in their eye. Interrupting them, I said "Hi Lesley."

She turned toward me and said, "Hi Guy. All is well I hope?" I answered, "Everything is great."

So many times before I wondered why I was here with the both of them. They would be doing all the talking. I would just sit back, listen, and enjoy their conversation. Still, It was wonderful to see them together again.

During the course of their conversation, I could not help but notice there was something very different about Lesley, and I was having a hard time reading her. I waited for the right opportunity to break into their conversation to ask her how she was feeling. In the past Lesley would share with us her own personal and family issues. She loved her children and always gave us the latest news about them. She also shared the latest news about her cancer. Previously she had told me her lung cancer was in remission and that she had never felt better. But, today I felt something was going on. Something wasn't right. Trying to find an appropriate way to ask again, how she was feeling, I simply asked if she were scheduled to see her doctor for a follow-up visit. Without hesitation, she said she had seen her doctor, and there was a concern about a relapse. There were signs and symptoms that her cancer had returned after a period of improvement.

Florence was extremely quiet, just staring at Lesley, not believing what she was listening too. I pressed on, cautiously, asking her what did that all mean? Lesley looked at Florence as she answered. You could not help but feel she was thinking of Florence and being very careful, choosing the right words that would not alarm her.

"Well, they tell me that the tumors seem to be growing."

Florence then glanced over at me, looking for a sign of assurance. I looked at her, and then back at Lesley.

Lesley continued, with an expression of confidence and said,

"They also said that they have a new drug that promises to shrink the tumors, and want me to start immediately on the treatment program."

Florence and I were at a loss for words for what seemed to be forever. But, Florence being the lady she is, only said, "Lesley, all of this will be behind you, just keep the faith and God will take care of the rest." Immediately, I remembered those exact words told to me, seven months ago, in the chapel, at St. Steven, by guess who – Lesley.

As we said our good bye's Lesley reached into her purse and pulled out an envelope. Smiling she gave it to Florence and said, "I hope you will enjoy this. It is your belated birthday present."

"Oh my," Florence said. "What are you doing? Can I open it now?"

Lesley said, "Of course, open it now. I hope you like what's in it."

Florence surprised, said, with tears in her eyes, "I can't believe this, how can I ever repay you?" "How, why?"

The gift was two tickets to see the Broadway play "Mamma Mia," and it included free parking.

Florence again, was at a loss for words, so was I!

"Lesley," Florence said, "How can we thank you?"

"You already have. The both of you gave me the most prized possession, your friendship. "May your birthdays always be as beautiful as your friendship has been to me."

Florence looked at me, smiling, that same grateful smile I've seen so often. Not until that moment did I realize the depth of the friendship between these two wonderful ladies.

"Friends are angels who lift us to our feet when our wings have trouble remembering how to fly."

- Author unknown

July 3, - Herceptin Treatment Continues

Today is Florence's scheduled Herceptin treatment. The treatment usually takes about ninety minutes, and so far Florence has tolerated the infusion well. The nurse continues to use Florence's vascular port to make it easier for her to receive the medicine. She has experienced very little discomfort, and there have been no side effects. When Florence first started Herceptin therapy treatment, the infusion took approximately thirty minutes. Her first treatment was on October 4. After fifteen treatments, one every week, the oncologist recommended a triple dosage of Herceptin. Not only because she was tolerating the medicine but also because she could take the treatment once per month rather than once per week. This was convenient for both of us. On January 31, she started the ninety-minute treatment and had no difficulty with the infusion. Now she has just four more to go. Her last is scheduled for September 24.

Florence's Herceptin therapy treatment is an involved process. The Herceptin infusion does not start immediately. First her vitals are taken and then a complete blood count (CBC) test is done. The CBC provides valuable information about the kinds and numbers of cells in her blood, especially red blood cells, white blood cells, and platelets. Basically, it is used for chemotherapeutic management. The outcome of the analysis is reviewed by the oncologist and based on sound results the oncologist gives the nurse technician the okay to start the procedure.

Today there is no known blood test to determine if cancer has spread beyond the lymph nodes upon the initial diagnosis. However, there is a tumor marker, CA27.29, used in the management of breast cancer patients that may indicate a systemic recurrence. The markers are proteins released by some tumor cells into the blood that may reflect the volume of tumors in the body. However, these proteins are also released by healthy tissues and may elevate for a nonmalignant reason.

The analysis has been performed four times since Florence has begun her chemotherapy treatments. Today, the nurse technician, will take another blood sample, and send it to the laboratory where different techniques are used to measure the level of the tumor marker. The analysis has been used to evaluate how well Florence has responded to her treatments and to check for the possibility of recurrence. The tumor marker levels have been measured over a period of time to see if the levels are increasing or decreasing. [74]Usually these serial measurements are more meaningful than a single measurement.

In Florence's Own Words

"July 18th: Started feeling less tired in the past week or so. Hopefully the Arimidex is settling down. I do need to have some caffeine everyday though, so need to keep track."

July 22nd: Dr. Diamond Radiologist Follow-up . . .
On April 23rd, Florence had finished her thirty-fourth day of radiation therapy. Part of her protocol was a follow-up visit with her radiation oncologist. Her radiation treatment, while it was truly inconvenient and the burns and the fatigue were no fun, overall it was completely doable. We both knew side effects would be an issue; though we were pleasantly surprised that she only had to deal with was a slight burning sensation, similar to a mild sunburn. Fatigue, however, was an issue.

Radiation therapy involves delivering X-rays to the location of her breast where Florence's cancer was removed. It is designed to destroy any cancer cells that may still be in the area. The therapy works within cancer cells to make them unable to multiply. The healthy tissue is then able to repair them selves in a way cancer cells cannot.

Florence took special care of her skin during the radiation therapy using a product called Aloe Vera Clear Gel. This product is both soothing and cool when applied. It provided an effective relief from her skin irritations, and minor burns. Also, it moisturizes the skin so that it would heal quickly. Florence found it perfect from the kind of damage that was caused by the radiation treatment.

Within two-months after Florence finished her radiation therapy, most of the side effects went away, however, fatigue was another matter. In Florence's case it was a distressing side effect of her cancer treatment. There is evidence that fatigue may persist for months or years after completion of successful treatments. For me, to see her often feeling tired, weak, and sometimes exhausted was always a concern. There were so many times I would find her in bed, during the day, and in those occurrences I felt so helpless and sad for her. This was not the Florence I knew.

I was aware that fatigue could have a profound negative effect on our quality of life. It could impact Florence's sense of wellbeing, her ability to perform her daily activities, and her relationship with family and our friends. And more than that, our own relationship would be tested. I understand there are a variety of factors that may contribute to fatigue. Her cancer treatments, low blood counts, sleep disruption, stress, poor nutrition, inactivity and medications. All can play a part.

Fatigue, as a result of cancer treatments, is not fully known or understood. It is a subjective experience, which means that only the individual experiencing it really knows how it feels. Cancer-related fatigue has been characterized as an overwhelming, whole-body tiredness that is unrelated to activity or exertion. Sleep or rest does not easily relieve it. The result is a decrease in energy and an increased need for sleep. There are other symptoms that describe fatigue; no pep; drained; a strong desire to stop and rest; a strong desire to lie down or sleep.

In Florence's Own Words

"Thursday July 24th: Herceptin today. Did well except for the last fifteen minutes. I started getting tired and not feeling well. My stomach hurt. Took a two-hour nap when I got home. Felt a little better after. Friday didn't get up till 10:45 AM, couldn't believe it. Felt pretty good after I got up. Took another little nap about 3:00 PM to 4:00 PM. We went to dinner with the kids, and I ate pasta, so I felt much better.

Thursday August 14th: Happy Birthday Dad! Herceptin today! Only two more to go after today! YEA! No problems just got really tired about half hour before I was done."

September 2nd – Mammogram . . .

Florence is sitting, waiting for her turn for a mammogram test. As always, I'm with her waiting also for the technician to escort her to the X-ray room. Sitting with her, I wondered if she realized that fourteen-months had gone by since she was last diagnosed. I asked her, "Florence, do you realize it's been fourteen-months since you started this journey?"

Yes, she answered. "I was just thinking of that. Wow, over a year has gone by already. Time flies!"

September is a special and busy month for Florence and me. On September 24th, she will complete her last Herceptin treatment for a total of twenty-six treatments. Tomorrow she will undergo a Mammogram, her third, and the following day a MUGA Scan, also her third, since being diagnosed in July. Even though we're somewhat excited that her treatments are coming to an end, it is sobering to contemplate that had effective treatments for breast cancer not existed, Florence would not be with me today. From the time she found her "Lump," last June till today, over a year later, Florence has had many frightening days. Even though I stood behind Florence when the doctors laid out the reality of her disease, there were times we had nothing positive to grab on to except hope and prayers. I remember discussing various treatment options, and between Florence and me, her surgeon, and her oncologist we decided on a treatment plan that would be best for her. She was to have six rounds of chemotherapy followed by thirty-three treatments of radiation including twenty-six sessions of Herceptin infusions, all of this over a fourteen-month period. Unfortunately, or fortunately, depends how you look at it, last June she also began hormonal treatments with a state-of-the-art drug called Arimidex. The Arimidex treatment program is one pill every day for five years. It will be May 2013 before she completes that treatment.

So, today is exciting for the both of us. It marks the last month of infusion treatments, blood test, etc., etc. Still, though, Florence will continue the Arimidex program and as a breast cancer survivor, will have a screening mammogram test at least annually. It will be necessary for Florence to perform monthly breast self-exams the same time every month. The more familiar she is with the contours and textures of her breast, and variations, the better off she will be. Having a regular clinical breast exam by her doctor will also be necessary. The object of these procedures is to be aware of any changes. This will be Florence's third mammogram procedure since last July.

After she completed the test, she came out of the room and sat next to me. "Wow," she said. "That hurt!"

"Hurt?" I said. I hated to hear her tell me she was in pain. The pain she endured over the fourteen-months from all the necessary procedures, and test, was an issue for me to contend with. I asked her,

"What do you mean it hurt?"

"You know that they place my breast on the mammography unit, and to get the best picture possible the technologist flattens my breasts on the platform. That hurts."

"You've had mammograms before; I don't remember you were complaining," I said.

Florence replied, "I don't understand why it is different this time. The pressure applied to the breast was incredibly painful. Maybe it's because of the surgery I had. The technician said she was sorry but explained it away as saying she needed to get the best view possible. At one point I said, "Hey, that really hurts. After three squishes later, she tells me to go get dressed and wait in the waiting room."

I knew she was hurting, so I placed my arms around her and assured her it would subside quickly.

I've read that the primary source of mammogram pain was the compression of the breast, and with about seventy-two percent of most women who rated mammogram pain; they said pain on a scale of one to ten was around a four. Many women say that the screening mammograms cause unnecessary anxiety and distress for seven out of eight women who are called back for more tests. However, many women find having regular breast screening very reassuring, knowing that it is very likely to pick up cancers at an early stage when treatments work best.

In regards to mammogram pain, I was reading the results of research done on screening mammograms in the journal, Radiology. If your pain tolerance is low, there is a new published study that found that applying four-percent lidocaine gel, an over-the-counter topical anesthetic, to the skin of the breasts and chest wall reduced mammogram discomfort during the test.

By far, our most stressful part of the mammogram experience is, waiting for the test results. We're always very frightened of recurrence. To go in and have the test, then to wait for several days or longer to get results is very stressful for us. Today, after the test the technologist said, "You will be happy to know that today's mammogram came up clean. We looked at each other, smiled, and said nothing. The technologist said, "See you next time at your routine annual mammogram."

In Florence's Own Words

"Thursday September 4th: Had Herceptin today. Got very tired at the very end. Lay around the rest of the day. ONE MORE TO GO, CAN'T WAIT!!!

Friday September 5th: Felt great all day today. I forgot to take my vitamins and Arimidex yesterday, I wonder if no Arimidex had anything to do with feeling good. Anyway, good day."

September 24th - Last Herceptin Treatment

Today is a milestone for Florence, so I started the day by visiting the chapel early in the morning. Kneeling down and trying to give my thanks to our Lord, I started thinking about this past year and how we both have arrived at this point of Florence's cancer journey. I know Florence will be as ecstatic, as I am that it is her last Herceptin treatment. I slowly moved my head around the chapel glancing at the wonderful friends sitting around me. It was then I realized just how many people care about Florence and me. I can't even begin to tell you how lucky we both are to have such amazing family and friends.

When I started my Christian walk, I gave myself to God all at once. In the beginning of my walk, I tried to explain the same maturity it had taken other Christians years to achieve. I suddenly found myself wholly changed. My soul, which had always been troubled, finally came to rest in a profound inner peace. I feel unable to express what is going on inside me right now. My former habits are seemingly forgotten. However, it has not always been that way. When I consider the blessings God has given Florence and me, and still continues to give, I feel ashamed. The incredible opportunities given to me I have abused. As I'm sitting here in the chapel, my mind starts to wonder and dwell on the "what ifs", problems with her Herceptin infusion, and the dreaded thought of recurrence. Will her cancer come back? "Stop," I said to myself. Why is my mind wondering toward the dark side? I need to recall my attention to God. I have to dwell in His presence immediately. Within seconds, and incredibly as it may seem, I immediately knew that Florence and I have very little control over whether or not the cancer returns, so why dwell on it? I need to focus on the things we can control in our lives, like our wonderful relationship together. Besides, today is a day of celebrating, being done with the Herceptin treatments.

After giving her friend, the receptionist, a hug, Florence was escorted, for the last time, into the chemo room. For the last time, she sat in a chemo chair, and for the last time she was connected to an infusion pole where the clear plastic bag containing the drug Herceptin hung. I was in the room with her as the nurse-technician methodically adjusted the valve that allowed the drug to flow down the clear tube and into her vascular port, and into her body, drip by drip. For the last time, I looked at the Herceptin bag assuring myself it was Trastuzumab

(Herceptin), and the right dosage of 409 mg, prescribed for Florence, and it was right. I kissed Florence and wished her good luck, and left the room. I sat in the waiting room, knowing I would be there for three-hours, the time it would take to empty the Herceptin bag. I opened my laptop to enter my notes about what was taking place as I did everyday. Weird as it may seem I kept thinking about the number of chemical drug's that had been infused into Florence's body over the past year. I had kept records of every appointment to include all of the drugs she had been taking. The following probably will not mean anything to you, the reader, and I wonder if it really means anything to me, now that it is over. Anyway, I have calculated the amount of chemo and Herceptin chemicals that was infused in her body.

Carboplatin = 3,018 mg or 3.018 grams or 0.106 ounces or 0.007 pounds

Taxotere = 762 mg or 0.762 grams or 0.027 ounces or 0.002 pounds

Herceptin = 7,153 mg or 7.153 grams or 0.252 ounces or 0.016 pounds

This does not include all of the secondary drugs injected each and every treatment, and does not include all of the blood removed from her body for diagnostics. That is another calculation I wish not to perform, and besides you're probably wondering why I would even add this to our story.

We're done with Herceptin treatments

Finally, after three-hours Florence came through the doors and into the waiting room. I immediately held up my hand, giving her the "OK" sign that indicated no more Herceptin treatments. It was over! She was done! She smiled at me, and we embraced. One more time, the receptionist, escorted her to the exit door and gave her one more hug. Through the tears, there were smiles. The receptionist didn't say much except to congratulate Florence and say her goodbyes. She had done this so many times. She knew how incredibly happy we both were, that the treatment journey was finally over. Yes, there were tears, tears of joy and yet, however, somber we may have been, thirteen-months did indeed go by. Thirteen incredible months! October, we will both meet with Florence's oncologist, Dr. Shroff. It will be her first follow-up consultation, including an up to date report on the status of her condition.

In Florence's Own Words

"September 24th: LAST ONE!!! Yabadabado!!! I'm done. Had no problems today, just same as always, a little tired. Took a long nap. Went to Guy & Janet's and they surprised me with dinner and balloons. It was really nice. Everybody was there but Clint. He was in San Francisco for Oracle."

October 23rd - Oncologist follow-up Appointment

Florence's first oncology consultation is creating significant stress, and we haven't arrived yet. The possibility of whether Florence's breast cancer could return is enough to frighten anyone, and that includes us. It is essential for me now, to be as confident as I can be. It is not the time to discuss "the what ifs." I reminded Florence she had done very well in all of her treatments, difficult as it was sometimes, the results have always been no signs of recurrence and/or progression of cancer.

More women are surviving breast cancer and living long and full lives. That, of course, is the good news. However, Florence still deals with long-term side effects of her chemotherapy and radiation treatments, and both of us still fear a recurrence. But, today was a day of happy tears. Wonderfully good news for the both of us! A clean report! Florence has been on her journey for fourteen-months and continues to do well. We both know the farther apart the appointments would be scheduled; the survival rate would increase. We are both looking forward to next August, another milestone. Twenty-four months, cancer free - complete remission. We pray this will be the case.

During our consultation, I raised the question as to when Florence's vascular implant port would be removed. I was thinking it could be removed within a couple of weeks. Not so! Dr. Shroff wanted to keep the port implant available as a precaution, in case there would be a recurrence. "How long?" I asked bewildered with what she just said.

She answered, "Guy, if we took the port out now, and then had, God forbid, a recurrence we would need to have Florence go through the surgery to put the port back in."

Again I asked, demonstrating some stress, "Doctor, how long before we can remove it?"

"I would like to keep it in for another twelve-months and flush it ever two-months. It will be important to keep the port from being contaminated with bacteria."

Listening to Dr. Shroff, I tried not to show any concerns, yet I was apprehensive with the whole notion of having the port-implant stay inside her breast. We have always felt comfortable with the doctor. She was always compassionate and went over in detail, all of Florence's issues. I looked at Florence to see if she felt confident in Dr. Shroff suggestion, and gave her a look of approval. Again, it would be Florence's decision to make. "Yikes," she said, "twelve more months before it's removed?" With a sense of stress she continued, "OK, I'll keep the port for the next twelve-months."

Although, deep down, I believed the doctor had made the right decision, it made me dwell on other reasons she may have had and would not tell us. Was Florence in that group of patients where greater than fifty percent, or higher, will have a recurrence? Was Dr. Shroff sending a message, in her own way, warning me of this likelihood? This reaction was very uncomfortable for me. Dr. Shroff has always given me as much time as I needed to ask detailed questions and to answer those questions regarding Florence's health issues. Asking her questions about the port, and why it should not be removed was answered logically, and straightforward. The only reason to keep the port within Florence was because of the recurrence concern. That does not mean a recurrence would take place. Florence has had the port implant for the last fourteen months, and obviously it turned out to be a blessing, since it lessened the pain of drug infusion. Another twelve-months should not make any difference, as long as it is maintained correctly.

After our meeting, we left feeling elated that Florence was indeed cancer free, and except for having to worry about the port maintenance for the next twelve-months, she must only be diligent with a physical health check-up every year by a health practitioner. This will include a yearly screening mammogram, and breast self-exams using the self-diagnostic technique.

Again, "What If?"

Florence emotions had been set aside during her cancer treatment. Now, they seem to becoming back, and again she felt overwhelmed with sadness, and anxiety. She was exhausted and tired all the time. It seemed apparent to me the lingering side effects of her treatments, was causing the fatigue; her body really needed a long rest. It's been a long time since she could really relax. Florence had been through a most difficult time. Cancer and all of the chemo, radiation, and

Herceptin treatments had invaded her body, and she had to make major life decisions throughout those last fourteen-months. The both of us really wanted to put the cancer behind us, but I could not help but notice that Florence was paying a lot of attention to her aches and pains, and looking for changes in her body. Dr. Shroff had said, "Florence, you have no signs of cancer" but can she really be sure? Sleeping, sometimes is an issue, and so many times we both coped with the emotional stress thinking, "what if?" All of these emotions, I've read, is normal. About seventy percent of cancer survivors are concerned about their cancer coming back. The fear of recurrence is a normal fear, and we both need to recognize that.

Cancer Survival – Recurrence . . .

According to the [75]American Cancer Society, the five-year survival rates for persons with breast cancer that is appropriately treated are as follows:

One-hundred percent for Stage Zero, one-hundred percent for Stage One, ninety-two percent for Stage Two A, eight-one percent for Stage Two B, sixty-seven percent for Stage Three A, fifty-four percent for Stage Three B, twenty percent for Stage Four.

Cancer survival rates are statistics that tell the percentage of people who survive for a specific amount of time. The five-year survival rate refers to the number of patients who live at least [75]five years after their cancer is found. It is based on research that comes from [76]information gathered on hundreds or thousands of people with cancer. As an example, five-year survival rate for prostate cancer is ninety-percent. That means that of all men diagnosed with prostate cancer, ninety of every one hundred were living five years after diagnosis.

Other types of survival rates that give [77]more specific information include: Disease-free survival rate and progression-free survival rate. Disease-free survival rate refers to the number of people with cancer who achieve remission. That means they no longer have signs of cancer in their bodies. Progression-free survival rate refers to the number of people who still have cancer, [77]but their disease isn't progressing. This includes people who may have had some success with treatment, but their cancer hasn't disappeared completely.

Act of Kindness - AOK

"If you want to lift yourself up, lift up someone else."
- Booker T. Washington

I'm not sure I would have talked about the "AOK's" let alone write about them if it were not for Florence's journey. The kind words, the kind deeds, from so many people was a wonderful statement of their generosity; that was generated deep in their hearts. It was indeed acts of kindness for Florence.

Wikipedia defines a random act of kindness as,

"A selfless act performed by a person or persons wishing to either assist or cheer up an individual. There will generally be no reason other than to make people smile, or be happier."

The above definition speaks volumes about Lesley Harris's character. Her AOK's toward Florence were compassionate, tender, and unselfish. When the discussion revolved around cancer, it was always about Florence's condition, her battle, her good times and her bad times. It never revolved around Lesley and her own issues with lung cancer. In Lesley's mind, this was about Florence, not about her. The lovely gifts she continued to give Florence, she considered small, but that was never the case in Florence's mind. They were indeed acts of kindness.

That wonderful morning in the Chapel, December, she opened my eyes toward what humankind is capable of doing. Think about it, how many times have we missed opportunities, losing sight of how easy it would be to warm someone's heart. How often have we found ourselves gossiping, finding fault, or talking negative about someone? Today, in our world, it seems acts of criticism, rather than acts of kindness are so prevalent toward those who disagree with us.

The Donut Man AOK

Even the smallest, most simple act of kindness can make the difference in people's lives in a very significant way. The Donut Man, I wrote about earlier, was a cancer patient who had a need to give back something, anything, to show his appreciation to the wonderful nurses and technicians at the Oncology Center for taking care of him during his battle with cancer. His AOK gift was a box of donuts delivered each week, not only to the nurse-technicians, but also to the cancer patients, including my wife, Florence.

It has happened to all of us. We're minding our own business and out of the corner of our eye we catch sight of an individual looking like he hasn't showered in months and holding out a cup begging for change from every passerby.

"It is futile to give money to beggars or poor people because most of the time they just spend that money on alcohol, etc." I have heard this more often than I like to hear.

The argument is, "Don't give him money he'll spend it on booze," others will say, "you'll never know what he spends it on." This argument, on both sides, has remained the same. However, I choose not to worry about it, although I would prefer the person spend it on what he had said he would spend it on.

When I give, I let go of that money and I don't think I have a right to suggest how the individual should use the funds. I think it's pretentious to give money with strings attached to those in need. My nephew, whom I love dearly, had a great idea. Buy food gift certificates. Keep them in your wallet so at the right time, you can give to those who are hungry and begging for food money. The reason is the person has to go to a shelter, or even McDonalds to turn in his gift certificate in exchange for food.

I believe Acts of kindness are really not difficult. We think of something to do, and we carry it out. It can be spontaneous or thought-out. Either way, when we give from the heart and enrich another person's life, it makes us feel good when we see our efforts contributing to someone else's well being.

Steven Grellet, a prominent French Quaker said,

"I expect to pass through life but once. If, therefore, there be any kindness I can show, Or any good thing I can do to any fellow being, let me do it now, as I shall not pass this way again."

Bread Angels AOK . . .

I would like to share an act of kindness that became a regular practice for me, and continues to give me great joy.

I was attending morning Mass at St. Stephen Chapel when a parishioner tapped me on my shoulder. This was the second tap on my shoulder; the first had been from Lesley Harris.

The parishioner apologized for the interruption, introduced himself, and asked if I would be willing to help out with providing and delivering food for the needy. He had seen me in the Chapel every Wednesday morning and was waiting for the opportunity to invite me to participate. He said, "Every Wednesday morning a group of my friends, and Chapel attendees, meet in one of the St. Stephen church rooms and pack bags with grocery items, mostly bread and pastries. The bags are then delivered to various needy homes in the community."

What a wonderful gesture, a wonderful act of kindness they were engaged in. Without hesitation, I said yes, I would be happy to join your group. Later, I would call this group the St. Stephen "Bread Angels."

Every Wednesday, after Mass, the Bread Angels meet and put together care packages for the needy. I know the folks who received these packages were delighted, especially the children, since the bags contained pastries. But I think it's not just what we give them that matters, it's what I see, the wonderful ray of light the Bread Angels give to the needy. This significant gesture of human kindness undoubtedly makes the recipient's world a much better place.

Harold Kushner, a prominent American rabbi said,

"When you carry out acts of kindness you get a wonderful feeling inside. It is as though something inside your body responds and says, yes, this is how I ought to feel."

Florence's Cancer Journey

"There are two ways to live your life . . . One is as though nothing is a miracle, the other is as though everything is a miracle."
- Albert Einstein

Someone once asked me; "How has cancer changed Florence?" This was a difficult question for me to answer. Florence has always been an ordinary woman with a wonderful life story. Her cancer journey, this trauma she endured, allowed her to look deeper for a new direction in her life. She would often say to me, "I don't know how to explain this feeling I have, but deep down I feel different inside." I tried to dig deeper into what she meant. She said that she never wanted cancer to invade her body, but since it had she never regretted the journey it has taken her on. Her journey has taught her a lot about herself and has reshaped her values and goals. She has a new perspective about life and relationships. She has lived through many challenges to her physical health, so it is easy for me to understand why she "feels different now." For many, a cancer experience is a potential launching pad to focus on meaningful life issues. Florence's cancer experience did change her. She is focusing on her core beliefs and has found ways to integrate her cancer experience with the rest of her life. I have to believe that God had prepared Florence for her cancer journey, even before she was diagnosed. The day that Florence was diagnosed, the Lord reached out His hand, - and held hers.

My Sacred Place

St. Stephen Community, through the leadership of Fr. John Bluett, has and continues to work hard to be messengers of faith, hope, and love. These virtues are experienced, not only at Mass on Sundays, but in the St. Stephen Chapel each morning. You can feel these emotions when you first enter the Chapel, and then look up to see the majestic Christ image gazing down upon the congregants.

For the past twenty-two months of Florence's journey, the chapel has been the focal point of my prayer and devotion. It is a room that has cultivated my sense of personal renewal, fostered by the feeling of being intimately aware of its inherent sacredness. During my visits each morning I learned that an active engagement with God was what was needed to grapple with the full mystery of my faith. It helped me keep hope alive when at times that was very difficult.

While I believe God is with us every step of our lives, I am convinced that a unique energy exists in the St. Stephen chapel, and I believe it is due to the active engagement of the participants. In other words, most of us wander through our lives oblivious to God's presence, to His calls to us. But through the act of entering the Chapel, we are in a sense saying, "Ok God, I am consciously here, I am ready to listen." Every morning this small group of people come to the Chapel, the reasons and their prayers are different from each other, yet they all share a common belief. There is a spiritual passion that occurs in the Chapel, and it surrounds these wonderful people who visit there. It flourishes in so many ways. As a result, I feel God's presence each, and every time I visit there.

It seems natural to me to say, "Hello God, I need your help!" It took me a long time to be able say those words, but with each such utterance it becomes a bit easier and I open up to Him more and more. I don't have it totally down yet, but I'm striving to be better at it. When I enter the Chapel, it seems as if I am instantly able to remove the egoist cloak I wear through life, and I can simply talk to Him. Formal prayers and deep meditations are not out of place here. To me it is a natural spot for God to exist, to listen, and to bring us hope, help, and understanding. It has and continues to be "My Special Place, - My Sacred Place."

"Take the first step in faith. You don't have to see the whole staircase, just take the first step."
- Martin Luther King, Jr.

Why Me? Why Her? Why?

Why did Florence, a wonderful wife, a good person, go through her journey with so much pain? Where was God in all of this? Why Florence, why me, why any of it? Anyone who has faced a serious illness, an accident, the potential or actual loss of a loved one, has grappled with this question. It seems God had ignored our cry for help? Has this happened to you? Were you angry and frustrated? Were you praying hard asking for His help and receiving nothing, no answer? No God, no response, only silence! He has not answered our prayers? Why? How come God allows bad things to happen, - and to good people?

From time to time on this journey, I too have made the plaintive cry, "Why me?" Worse, when I made that initial, heartfelt "plea" to God, when I needed His comfort and assurance, He was nowhere to be found, as if He didn't exist. But then; if God doesn't exist, to whom am I crying out to? If God has no place in my heart, why is my first instinct to seek His comfort and grace? Clearly, I must believe there is a God out there who hears me, and I'm hopeful He will respond.

Suffering exists. The first Noble Truth of the Buddha ("Life is suffering"). I know it causes problems for many of us in our approach to God, and I don't think scripture does much to explain the cause of suffering. However, scripture does promise that God is with us and will help us get through the pain if we but only ask for that help and believe it will come.

Suffice it to say, when Florence's illness struck, when the awful truth was made so abundantly clear to us both, I was in no mood for abstract or theoretical discussions about suffering, God, or noble truths. I wanted – I needed – help, relief from the terrible pain that gnawed at my insides. When you're in the thick of suffering, it is the suffering that matters, not its causes. When I first entered the world of cancer I was filled with questions, frustration, anger, and sadness. Cancer is horrible, painful, and terrifying – it was the unseen enemy that had invaded Florence's body. It is this type of experience that brings to your mind so many personal thoughts about God! At least it did for me. Florence's pain and suffering indeed influenced my relationship with God. It did not distance me from God as it does to so many people. It produced a new dimension in my understanding of God's ways. "Why me?" I think I will leave that subject to the scholars.

Now, after twenty-months, Florence and I remain haunted by fears that the disease will return. I recognize that those fears are normal, that the word "remission" can seem awfully temporary next to the cancer itself. However, it still makes Florence and me anxious, and that anxiety only intensifies as the next check-up nears, or with the news of a friend being diagnosed with this disease. I also know, however, that there will be a day, when we will no longer be preoccupied with thoughts of breast cancer recurrence.

Florence's journey began with a scheduled biopsy of the lump she'd found in her breast months earlier. I will never forget that day. I was waiting for her to come out of the operating room. It was a day. I was truly overwhelmed by everything going on around me, like an animal captured and thrown into a cage, and felt I was losing control. In many ways, I was the typical male, imagining myself able to "fix" whatever problem ailed her. Only I couldn't, and that feeling of helplessness was beginning to consume me.

I left the building, leaving her in the hands of her doctors. The biopsy, one of the most significant events in Florence's life, would take place without me. As I was leaving, something penetrated my inner heart and took possession over me. It was something that, to this day, I have a hard time describing. It was a must, almost a compulsion, to find sanctuary in a church, a sacred place. I was in need of help.

In an irony that escaped me at the time, I essentially was conceding that, in the same way that I had no control, that I could not help Florence, neither could anyone help me.

Even as I pen these words that same male ego – the ego that tucked tail and ran during the biopsy – is trying very hard not to divulge any more about my "weakness," about the terror I experienced that day. But it is precisely because the ego betrayed itself for what it is that I push on, that I record these words, that I acknowledge something more than me was needed that day. I literally cried all the way to the church. I cried in the church, and I cried all the way back to the doctor's office. I felt so vulnerable. I was a man, an athlete, a successful businessman; a father and grandfather several times over, and I was supposed to be strong, to handle this as I'd handled every other challenge that had come my way. Understandably, I didn't like what was happening to me. That day I officially joined what I've come to euphemistically call the "Crier's Club."

What compelled me to visit the church? I just as easily could have visited the nearby Denny's or sought refuge in the reassuring words of our children or a friend. But that something – that "still, inner voice" – drove me to a church, specifically, St. Margaret Mary Catholic Church. Was it faith that drove me to visit the church? Did I already have the faith, in God, to cope with this new event in our lives?

Most of us think we can turn to God for help. When we seek God's help, however, we do so without really expecting to give up anything of ourselves or even with the expectation that must change anything in our lives. We think we can add spirituality the way we do a new kitchen to our homes – as if it's a simple shopping cart transaction.

But if God were so easily acquired, if our prayers were so easily answered, would there be war, murder . . . cancer? Picture the millions upon millions of prayers that each day were issued in the name of "God" and then imagine the suffering that continues to plague us all. Have we eliminated disease, have we brought peace to this fragile world, has our beloved, the one for whom we care so deeply - has she been freed of the cancer attacking her body? Have we really brought God into our human existence?

I came to see that there must be a turning point in our lives and that that turning point for me, the change I needed to make, was to bring God back into my life.

"My Awakening to Faith"

With the passage of time and the grace of God, we came to recognize the blessings that resulted from Florence's breast cancer diagnosis. We saw that the experience brought everyone that was a part of our lives closer together. For me, it was an experience that led me to make important changes in my life. The biggest and the most important was to reinvent my belief system, to define my faith in God. It wasn't easy, and it took a long time to honestly grasp it. There have been so many times I would watch and listen to family members or close friends, trying to understand where their faith came from. For some, it seemed easy, and I was envious. I wanted to copy their belief system.

We all would agree that faith is the belief in a higher power or being. But where did that faith that belief in God originate? For me, it wasn't enough to hear the blanket statement, "I believe in God." I needed more than that.

Recently Florence and I have traveled up and down the U.S. and Canadian Rockies, marveling at their awesome beauty. The lush valleys and snow-capped peaks, the glaciers and glacial lakes; the sheer wonder and majesty of nature has always left us breathless. But more than that, it has prompted me to ponder their Architect, to ponder God.

There have been times, late at night, when she and I would lay outside on a warm blanket gazing up at a starlit night. We'd compete to see who would spot the first meteorite traveling across the sky. And as we stared up into that inky blackness, into the Milky Way and its millions and millions of stars, we could not help but wonder about its origins. Nature, I believe, does bring us closer to the essence of God. How can it not? The profound beauty and awesomeness provides a positive argument for the existence of God.

My several mentions of "God" may lead you to conclude that I do have faith; that by speaking of nature's beauty I am convinced of His presences and His role as Architect and Master. But it is not easy. Yes, I have faith, but a conscious relationship with God takes time, and at least for me it has unfolded over time, spurred both by Florence's cancer as well as those Rocky Mountain nights.

So you might ask, if God exists for you, what is the problem? I'm hopeful all of this will make sense to you, and more than that I'm hopeful it will make sense to me. Please don't read this as one who is trying to postulate his newfound faith. Far from being a spiritual lecture, it is in reality my spiritual confession or, perhaps, an announcement of my spiritual rebirth. It is a testament to what I have experienced.

"Very truly I tell you, no one can see the kingdom of God without being born again."
- John 3:3

Faith is antithetical to the human ego, which demands empirical evidence. By definition, faith says it should be enough to say, God is. That God created all things, including us. But many of us want physical evidence. After the crucifixion of Jesus, scripture tells us, Thomas, one of Jesus' twelve disciples, would not believe unless he saw Jesus. When Jesus appeared before Thomas, he said:

"Because you have seen me you have believed, blessed are those who have not seen and yet believe." - John 20:29

This is a profound statement – "Blessed are those who have not seen and yet believe."

Believing what we did not see; yet in our hearts we know it is true - that is faith!

Someone once compared faith to the wind. He said you couldn't see the wind, or hear the wind unless it blows against something. You can only feel the wind when it touches our skin or rustles the trees. Faith is like that wind. We cannot see what we believe in, and we cannot hear what we believe in unless we open our eyes to the truth. Faith was an acceptance of what I couldn't see, but I could feel it deep within my heart. It didn't jump out at my innermost self, no matter how much I practiced spirituality or how good I was to someone else. Faith came from outside of me and then found its way into my heart. AND, it wasn't how strong my faith was, but who my faith was in. This I believe happened to me.

Mercifully, cancer didn't mean the end of Florence's life, as we both initially feared. If anything, her journey opened my eyes to the word of God, reaching my mind, heart, and knowing and understanding it. In my case hearing and perceiving the testifiers of the gospel, the writers of the sacred book, the prophets, and the apostles have helped the renewal of my faith. Yet, something had to kick-start the process. For me, it was that first week of July. It was overshadowed by fears of losing Florence, as well as all the other fears associated with that loss. At the same time, it was a week of the usual structured human existence: Mammogram on Tuesday, Sonogram on Thursday, and Biopsy on Friday. That Friday was an eventful day for me, and certainly for Florence. The visit to St. Margaret Mary would start a 24-month journey of renewing my faith. As I said, I cannot describe what happened, but I was indeed touched, and from that day forward there would be daily, early-morning visits to St. Stephen chapel. The chapel visits provided me with the spiritual illumination, which came to me from hearing, listening and reading. Reading is a form of hearing. It is a sort of hearing with your eyes. When I'm listening to the gospel or the readings of the scriptures, I do not allow myself to focus on the priest, the preacher or the lector. Though the person speaking may be eloquent and articulate, or he/she may be stammering, and his voice may be disagreeable, it is not so much the delivery of the message itself but the word of God itself.

During this time, I reached out to my Savior, and asked Him to walk beside me. I felt a peace come over me as though someone was there. There wasn't anyone around, but I just sense that everything would be okay. I know now I could not have carried the burdens of those incredible fears, the anxieties by myself. I learned He would guide me, and keep me strong throughout Florence's journey. He helped me hold on to my faith, even in the worst of times, and I would simply say, "Stay with me."

From the depth of my soul, I am so grateful for this journey.

"Amazing Grace, how sweet the sound, that saved a wretch like me . . . I once was lost but now am found, was blind, but now, I see . . ."
- John Newton

Letter To My Husband

In Florence's Own Words

"Dear Guy,

First of all, my thoughts and feelings for you are so "big" that I can't even come up with the right words for them. So, I simply say, I love you more and more everyday and can't even imagine that we could be anything else but "one." I know the kids and grandkids would say jokingly, "Mom/grandma, you're giving Dad/grandpa a big head, and we already have a problem with him," as they laugh. But we both know what they are really thinking. They all love you so much.

I know some will have a hard time believing some of the things I will say in this letter, and that's probably why I never shared these thoughts with anyone - even you, until now.

Strange as it may sound, I believe my cancer diagnosis was the first of many gifts, and I thank God for those gifts every day.

For example, when my treatments first started I remember overhearing something on the television about how "one out of every three woman will get breast cancer." Well, I did the math and counting my sisters, Beverly and Theresa, it turned out that I ended up being the "winner." But I honestly felt something so comforting knowing it was me and not Beverly or Theresa. I know I would have had a horrible time seeing and coping with them going through anything to do with cancer. I immediately thanked God.

The second gift was this overwhelming sense of gratitude for being given this 'opportunity' for personal growth. I know this is the part you had a problem with. How can you be grateful for getting cancer? Well, it's just a matter of fact. When I was told I had breast cancer, and it was very bad, my first thoughts were of you and our children. It was gut wrenching. How do I tell them? How do I tell them not to worry? How do I tell them I'm okay with it - well as okay as I could be - and that whatever happens I WILL BE OK! Of course all of this was one emotion running into another emotion, and we all got through this part together. I do not know what I would do without you or them; you all, are my heart.

I remember again the first day going into the Florida Cancer Institute. After the first shock of seeing that sign with the word 'cancer' emblazoned across it and knowing that I was the person for whom that sign was intended, it turned out that after that initial shock, something very special happened to us both. When we stepped off of the elevator onto the third floor, the first thing we saw was a beautiful painting of a crane. We both looked at each other and couldn't believe it. What a wonderful beginning, the Bird of Peace welcoming us. Wow!

After my first Chemo session, we walked out to the hallway and noticed some motivational pictures adorning the walls. We spent some time reading some of them. You motioned me over to one. It read, "I believe life is a journey and my destination will be blessed." For whatever reason, those words sent a shiver down my spine. Someone, I thought, is watching over us. I just knew it, first the crane, now this? Then we proceeded to look at some of the others. I don't remember any other words passing between us, but we both knew we had to write some of these wonderful statements down. I still have them.

"I believe God carries my heart"
"I believe in faith and family"
"I believe in the healing power of prayer"
"I believe in God, family and friends"
"I believe I have more to do"

We both have seen beautiful photos with sayings at other hospitals but none like these. I felt every one of those statements was a message for me, and I tried to keep them in my heart from then on. To this day I believe in every one of them and that in their own way they leant me strength during that long journey.

Even though I know you already talked about this in your book, I have to mention the crane again. Our first introduction to this bird was after Barbara passed away. Your stories, Jim's stories, and others were too crazy not to be true. It's very hard to explain to people, but we all know in our hearts they were messages sent from above. I thought, and even talked to Barbara so often during this time. I never heard her, but I knew she was listening. I felt such a bond with her; especially knowing she had breast cancer and knew what I was feeling. I remember Jim sending me a note about the Crane that said, "Barbara was very conscious about her long neck. I used to kid her about it. Early in our relationship she said to me, "Ha, little do you know, in the Far East, birds with long necks, are, a thing of beauty. When you think of me think of one of those beautiful birds, the "Crane".

Once the initial emotional stress of the cancer diagnosis and those early treatments settled down a bit, I began to understand that I was being given an opportunity and I needed to do something about it. I was going through the biggest part of this nightmare, but when I saw someone else in those "chemo, lazy boy chairs" who looked so much worse off than me, I had to do something about it. Some of these people were even there by themselves, one having to catch a bus home by herself. My heart ached for these people. okay, I thought, just say hello, and maybe start a little conversation, or just smile and give them a look that says, "Isn't this a drag?" I did just that, and it worked. I got so many expressions of gratitude and smiles, and comments like, "We do have something in common, don't we?" And I thought, "Wow, this really is a gift. I just helped someone in such a small way, but it really made me feel good, and even helped ease a little of the rest of my three-and-a-half-hour treatments. We were sharing something, maybe our humanity or our suffering. We were saying, through those smiles and small gestures, "We aren't alone. Others are fighting right alongside us."

Perhaps the most valuable gift of all is my newfound appreciation for life itself. I look at it so differently now. If I can be there anytime for anyone who might need a hand, I will do my best to be there. I now understand what someone goes through with pain and fear, especially the fear of the unknown. I know my journey through this was not even close to what others are going through, or will go through. I've always loved life, but now every day really is a gift.

Still another gift: Guy, you go to Mass every morning now. You were given a gift during this time, but I'm not sure you consider all of this has been "an opportunity." We love each other more now than we ever have. We've always had a great relationship, but we didn't get this far without ups and downs in our lives, like any other couple. The song by Josh Groben, "You Lift Me Up," says so much of what you have done for me during this whole venture.

As I mentioned in my cancer diary, the kids and grandkids were unbelievable. From seeing the saddest looks on all of their faces, to some of the funniest comments I have ever heard, they all shined. It was almost as if the cancer gave all of us permission to be more honest and authentic than we had ever before dared. I'll never forget Clint's comment when I finally lost the last wisps of hair and became totally bald. "Mom, why don't you get a magic marker and have everybody sign your head?"

I loved all the humor, hugs and caring that you, the kids, and grandkids showed me throughout this trial. I know I was cranky and wasn't in the best moods all the time, but I still felt so loved by all of you during that time.

Getting back to the hair, the following meant so much to me. Don't know who wrote it, but it is very powerful.

ATTITUDE

There once was a [79]woman who woke up one morning, looked in the mirror, and noticed she had only three hairs on her head. Well," she said, "I think I'll braid my hair today." So she did and she had a wonderful day.

The next day she woke up, looked in the mirror, and notice that she had only two hairs on her head.

"Hmm," she said, "I think I'll part my hair down the middle today." So she did and she had a grand day.

The next day she woke up, looked in the mirror, and noticed that she had only one hair on her head.

"Well," she said, "Today I'm going to wear my hair in a pony tail." So she did and she had a fun, fun day.

The next day she woke up, looked in the mirror, and noticed that there wasn't a single hair on her head.

"YEA!" she exclaimed, I don't have to fix my hair today!"

ATTITUDE IS EVERYTHING

Be kinder than necessary, for [80]everyone you meet is fighting some kind of battle. Live simply, Love generously, Care deeply, and speak kindly, leave the rest to God.

Life isn't about waiting for the storm to pass... It's about learning to dance in the rain.

Looking back at the log I kept, I think about each of those incredible days. Some brought joy and sweet memories, others a sense of shame and regret. When life comes right at you and stares you in the face, you can't help but think of the past. Of course, there are things you wish you could change and redo, but you have to put those behind you and be grateful for where you are now in your life. I am in a beautiful place right now.

My sisters, brothers, and their spouses and families, and your sister Jocelyn and her family were so supportive during this time. Talk about a loving family. The emails, phone calls, prayers and love they showed were amazing. I remember what Sally Field said when winning an acting Oscar. "You like me, you really like me." It got a big laugh. I feel the same way, "They like me, they really like me."

The final gift was our friendship with Lesley Harris, who in many ways gave more to you and me than anyone could imagine. We both know and believe she was an angel sent to us. Those times we were together, the first thing I saw was a beautiful smile on her face, and then we would hug each other, and continue to hug for a few seconds more. Those wonderful moments

I think of all the time. I can't exactly explain the feeling, but it's like she is saying, "Everything is going to be okay Flo," and I felt it was. I only wish I could have done something more for her.

I'll never forget when we were talking one day, after she found out she didn't have much time left, and we started crying, talking about life, her daughters, - and time. She stopped in the middle of our conversation and said, "Flo, I have not had a problem since this started accepting the fact that it is my time. In fact, I thank God for giving me the time to spend with my children, Alexa and Amanda, and trying to help them understand what is going on. I want them to know I will not be here physically, but I will always be with them. I was blessed also to be able to have the time to get some things in order, and to say my good-bye's to the people I love. You know; I could have been taking the girls to school and gotten in an accident and been taken then, or worse, could have lost my girls. So we have to accept what life gives us and be grateful for it."

What a fighter, I thought to myself, what a spiritual person she is. Her words are captured inside me and will be with me forever.

I keep thinking of how positive she was, and I never heard one word from her where she was feeling sorry for herself, or questioning "Why me?" I really hope someday I'll be able to pass on the gift she gave me.

We also were blessed with meeting Lesley's brother Marc and his wife Janine. They are the most wonderful people, and now we are friends with them. They are so giving. I don't think their family would have gotten through all those trying times without Janine. She came for one visit after Lesley's news, and never left till Lesley passed. She was surely Lesley's angel during that time. She was able to take care of all the necessary things that the family could not handle while she was there. We are so lucky to have really grown to love Janine and Marc.

I have learned so much from this journey; it wasn't fun, but life is not all fun, and if we can come away with something good and special, and we were given that opportunity to do so, we have to be very thankful for it. I really do believe it was a gift from God, that He awakened something in me, in my life. God doesn't decide one day to say "OK Florence, I'm going to give you cancer today". He does not work that way. I never once asked, "why me?" I know God was right there with me from the day I first heard those three words that no one ever wants to hear, "You have Cancer". If you know God, you know He would never wish anything like this on you. He is there to help you get through it, and I feel sure He feels the same pain we feel. "I love God."

I also cannot thank enough; all the family who continued to send their thoughts and prayers to us during our journey. They meant everything to me - another wonderful gift!

I am so overwhelmed by the sheer volume of the life I have lived. I have always been so fortunate to have you and the family we have, the biggest gift of all. Now you all stand out like 3D; you are bigger than life. I love you all so much.

There aren't enough words to thank our children and grandchildren, Guy Anthony, Janet, Clint, Vickie, Joshua, Jordan, Jessica and Amanda, for making our journey so caring and compassionate. They truly gave me the strength I needed to get through this venture. I couldn't stand it when anyone of them looked even a little sad, so inside I tried hard not to do anything that would make them feel that way.

I loved all the humor from every one of them, and there was a lot of it, Thank God! From small funny comments, to big funny comments, to the grandkids putting on little shows and entertaining me, to playing games and laughing almost the whole time we played. There are to many times too begin to write them down. Anyway, we were given a huge blessing, a gift from God by having them a part of our journey. God bless them.

I couldn't have been more blessed than to have my brothers and sisters, and their families with me on my cancer journey. Their cards, their emails, their visits, and their phone calls, I will never forget. The little ones were absolutely wonderful. The sweet cards they sent were so awesome. I'll never forget once when little Skylar sat down next to me, put her arm around me and said, "How are you doing Aunt Florence?" I said, "I'm doing pretty good Skylar." She looked at me with a big smile and said; "I knew that because I say a prayer for you every night." She then reached over and gave me a kiss. Man, I had a hard time holding those tears back. So, as I said before, who could ask for anything more? I love all of them so much, and I thank them again. God bless them all.

The gift of friends! Bob and Carol Baratta were so wonderful, as always. Just knowing that Bob was there for you at any time, settled my worrying. He was so great, Guy, with the calling, humorous emails, and getting doctors he knew to confirm some of the things we were concerned about. I also knew Carol was there for me anytime I might need her. Our trip to visit them in Maine shortly after my diagnosis was amazing. What a lift they were, and still are. From the moment, we walked into their house, and they had that bottle of OPUS waiting for us, till the time we left, was absolutely wonderful.

Of course, I started with the tears, then the wine, then the laughs. They are so much more than special.

There are so many others, Father George and Father John, their caring and hugs had such a significant spiritual impact on me. Dr. Jan, who was such a great help to us, and her sister Ellen. God remembers when they were young some forty years ago. It's hard to believe Jan is a doctor now with three children, and Ellen also has three children. I love those girls. Coach Stitch and Jacque, Diane, Carolyn (breast cancer survivor), Gil, with his call to you all the way from Bahrain when he heard the news, Tommy and his wife Kathy, (breast cancer survivor), Heather, our amazing group of high school buddies, Sister Pauline, and so many more that we thankfully have. I can't thank them enough for being there for us.

So by now I'm sure you understand the opportunity I was given. It reminds me of when we went to see the movie "Evan Almighty", and some of the quotes from that movie.

"Let [81]me ask you something. If someone prays for patience, do you think God gives him or her patience? Or does he give them the opportunity to be patient?

If he prayed for courage, does God give him courage, or does he give him opportunities to be courageous?

If someone prayed for the family to be closer, do you think God zaps them with warm fuzzy feelings, or does he give them opportunities to love each other?"

I don't think I would ever want to get this particular "opportunity" again. But now I do look forward to every day I wake up to see what opportunity today will bring me.

Thank you again for being so kind, compassionate, and loving, always telling me I was pretty and looked nice.

Guy, I would never have gotten through this without you. There were days when I looked at you and knew what you were thinking and feeling, but you always kept your pain inside, and worried only about me. The times you just held my hand, or put your arms around me, meant so much to me. We didn't have to say a word. I just knew how much you loved me and how much I loved you. We're so very blessed to have something very special together. Always!

I love you, Florence"

Epilogue

On May 31st, Florence was rushed to the hospital with severe flu-like symptoms. The diagnosis was a blood related bacterial infection caused by her vascular port implant, the port that had been used for chemotherapy drug infusion. The port was to be removed in September but because of her emergency diagnosis it was surgically removed immediately. Florence was released from the hospital five days later; the infection gone.

On August 13th, she officially became a twenty-month survivor.

Florence's cancer may be in remission, but the cancer war continues to be waged on many fronts. On March 8, Lesley Harris (Lady in Black) passed away. She died as she had lived - courageously fighting to the end.

This wonderful angel has indeed touched our lives. She will forever be missed, but I know in the right time, Florence and I will meet Lesley again. We will ALL MEET Lesley again, and she'll make us laugh and she'll greet us with that contagious smile, and say "Welcome Home."

Well done Lesley, for you have made a difference in peoples lives. God bless you and your family.

Five years later, on August 13th, Florence officially became a Five Year Survivor. May 9th, nine months later, she completed her Arimidex hormonal therapy treatment. Three months later, August 13th, Florence completed six years of cancer treatments. Officially, she became a "Six Year Cancer Survivor . . ."

Notes

[1] Emails and Phone Calls
http://www.wherepeacefulwaters.com/readings/26_guards.htm

[2] The Crane
http://www.sos-walk.org/sos/crane.htm

[3] The Crane
http://www.artofzenyoga.com/?page_id=27

[4] The Crane
http://smarterthanmatt.blogspot.com/2008_12_01_archive.html

[5] The Crane
http://www.dailykos.com/story/2013/08/06/1229198/-Aug-6-1945-
Hiroshima-and-Sadako-and-the-Thousand-Paper-Cranes

[6] Learning About Cancer
http://www.healthtipsforwomen.net/facts-about-breast-cancer/
what-is-breast-cancer-and-what-part-of-breast-is-cancer-found-in.

[7] Learning About Cancer
http://www.oregonsurgical.com/surgery_oncology.htm

[8] Ten Days of Tests
http://www.apollohealthcity.com/Pet_Scan/cancer.htm

[9] Ten Days of Tests
http://www.healthcentral.com/breast-cancer/c/78/143111/carboplatin/

[10] August 13th - Time For Surgery
http://melanoma.surgery.ucsf.edu/conditions--procedures/
sentinel-lymph-node-biopsy.aspx.

[11] Living With Uncertainty
What is a breast cancer grade? - Diagnostic Biopsy
http://www.sharecare.com/question/what-is-breast-cancer-grade

[12] Living With Uncertainty
http://www.medhelp.org/posts/Breast-Cancer/
biopsy grade/show/1158063.

[13] Cancer Staging
Cancer 101: Cell Grades and Differentiation,
http://www.baymoon.com/~gyncancer/library/weekly/aa062001a.htm

[14] Cancer Staging
http://www.cancer.org/cancer/breastcancer/detailedguide/
breast-cancer-staging?level
http://www.cancer.org/cancer/breastcancer/detailedguide/
breast-cancer-staging?level

[15] Cancer Staging
Stages of Breast Cancer, http://breasthealthhouston.com/
content.asp?secnum=14

[16] Cancer Staging
http://ucanhealth.com/topics/?T=breast_cancer_stages
http://flaxhullignans.com/stagesbc.php

[17] Cancer Staging
http://answers.yahoo.com/question/
index?qid=20060703220017AAOQmU3

[18] Cancer Staging
How is Breast Cancer Staged - uCan Health - A Source of ..,
http://ucanhealth.com/topics/?T=breast_cancer_stages
http://ucanhealth.com/topics/?T=breast_cancer_stages

[19] Cancer Staging
Breast Cancer, http://www.cancer.org/cancer/news/breast-cancer

[20] Cancer Staging
http://www.sharecare.com/question/types-of-breast-cancer

[21] Cancer Staging
http://www.whereincity.com/medical/topic/cancer/diseases/
breast-cancer-46.htm

[22] Oncotype DX Test
http://www.healthsearches.org/Categories_of_Q&A/Diagnosis/1326.php

[23] Florence Treatment Protocol
http://www.cancer.org/cancer/%20livercancer/detailedguide/
liver-cancer-treating-chemotherapy

[24] Florence Treatment Protocol
http://www.ncbi.nlm.nih.gov/pubmedhealth/PMHT0009459/
http://chemocare.com/chemotherapy/what-is-chemotherapy/
cancer-cells-chemotherapy.aspx

[26] Florence Treatment Protocol
http://www.breastcancer.org/treatment/targeted_therapies/
herceptin/side_effects

[27] Alternative Treatments
http://www.quack-watch.org/01QuackeryRelatedTopics/altwary.html

[28] Alternative Treatments
Science meets alternative medicine - Columbia University in ..,
http://www.columbia.edu/cu/21stC/issue-3.4/walker.html

[29] Alternative Treatments
http://www.quack-watch.org/01QuackeryRelatedTopics/altwary.html

[30] Alternative Treatments
CSCT, Inc. - Federal Trade Commission,
http://www.ftc.gov/opa/2003/02/csct.shtm

[31] Alternative Treatments
http://www.ftc.gov/opa/2004/02/csct.shtm

[35] Alternative Treatments
http://fitnessmagazineinfo.blogspot.com/2005/09/
american-health-and-fitness-magazine.html

[36] Alternative Treatments
http://www.healthrecoverygroup.com/pmp/index.htm

[37] Paranormal Events
http://www.internationaleducationgroup.net/
Schools/SchoolProfile.aspx?id=235

[38] Paranormal Events
http://www.medjugorje.org/overview.htm

[39] Florence and Robert Urich
http://www.spenser.de/roberturich-com/page2.html

[40] Saint Peregrine - The Cancer Saint
http://www.theworkofgod.org/Saints/Lives/Peregrin.htm

[41] Saint Peregrine - The Cancer Saint
St. Peregrine, http://www.stperry.org/perry.htm

[42] Saint Peregrine - The Cancer Saint
http://www.oocities.org/heartland/meadows/4798/novena.html

[42] Saint Peregrine - The Cancer Saint
http:www.oocities.org/heartland/meadows/4798/novena.html

[43] I'm Learning How to Pray
http://www.catholicdoors.com/courses/howtopray.htm

[44] I'm Learning How to Pray
http://www.catholicdoors.com/courses/howtopray.htm

[45] The Dreaded Side Effects
Managing eating problems caused by surgery, radiation, and ..,
http://www.cancer.org/treatment/survivorshipduringandaftertreatment/
nutritionforpeoplewithcancer/%20nutritionforthepersonwithcancer/
nutrition-during-treatment-manage-eating-probs

[46] November 7th - Heart Palpitations
Heart Rhythm Changes (Arrhythmias) - Managing Side Effects .., http://
chemocare.com/chemotherapy/side-effects/heart-rhythm-changes.aspx

[47] December 4th - Shingles
Shingles Herpes zoster Malaysia- Virue Kayap Acupuncture ..,
http://www.oocities.org/shingersherbs/

[48] December 4th - Shingles
Prayer Center | Prayer for my wife. | Streaming Faith,
http://www.streamingfaith.com/index.php/prayer/viewthread/24483/

[49] Chemo Brain
http://www.riversideonline.com/health_reference/Cancer/CA00044.cfm

[50] Chemo Brain
http://www.drlarrylachman.com/people/chemobrain.php
http://www-cgi.cnn.com/HEALTH/library/CA/00044.html

[51] Chemo Brain
http://www.drlarrylachman.com/people/chemobrain.php

[52] Chemo Brain
http://www.chemobraininfo.org/IntroChemo.htm

[53] Chemo Brain
www.learnenglishbest.com/what-is-in-a-name.html

[54] Chemo Brain
www.singlec.com/scnendor2.htm

[55] Radiation Treatment - The Journey
http://www.imaginis.com/mammography/
mammography-and-imaging-after-breast-cancer-surgery.

[56] Radiation Treatment - The Journey Continues - March 5th - Mammogram Tests
http://www.breastcancer.org/symptoms/testing/
types/mammograms/after_surgery

[59] Good News
J. RESTREPO EQUIPHOS
http://www.equiphos.com/en/noticiaDetalle.php?id=25

[60] Good News
Frederick Regional Health System
http://www.fmh.org/body.cfm?id=12&action=detail&ref=41

[61] Good News
http://www.mail.archive.com/pituitarychat@groups.msn.com/
msg04661.html
http://www.mail.archive.com/pituitarychat@groups.msn.com/
msg04661.html

(62) Good News
http://www.mail-archive.com/pituitarychat@groups.msn.com/
msg04661.html

[63] Good News
http://en.wikipedia.org/wiki/Background_radiation

[64] Good News
www.equiphos.com/en/noticiaDetalle.php?id=25

[65] Bad Hair Day
http://www.acco.org/Information/drugsgeneraleffects.aspx
http://www.ucsfhealth.org/education/autologous_transplant_guide/
blood_counts_and_transfusions/
http://www.hematology.org/patients/blood-basics/5222.aspx

[67] CA27.29 - Tumor Marker
http://www.doctorslounge.com/oncology/labs/ca27-29.htm

[68] May 9th - Florence Starts Hormonal Treatments
http://antibiotics.emedtv.com/search.html?searchString=treatment%
20of%20uti&page=23

[69] May 9th - Florence Starts Hormonal Treatments
http://www.netdoctor.co.uk/cancer/medicines/arimidex.html

[70] June 12, – Oncologist Appointment - June 16th - DEXA Scan
http://www.white-wilson.com/imaging/imaging_womens.htm
http://healcon.com/healthbook/healthtopic/
osteopenia_AwN3LwuwZGEuKmxlAQZ=.htm

[72] June 12, – Oncologist Appointment - June 16th - DEXA Scan
http://en.m.wikipedia.org/wiki/Bone_density

[73] July 3, - Herceptin Treatment Continues
http://www.medhelp.org/posts/Breast-Cancer/CA-19-blood-test/
show/467858

[74] July 3, - Herceptin Treatment Continues
http://www.medhelp.org/posts/Breast-Cancer/CA-19-blood-test/
show/467858

[75] October 23rd - Oncologist follow-up Appointment -
Cancer Survival – Recurrence
http://www.advocatehealth.com/bromenn/blank.cfm?ID=70
http://www.advocatehealth.com/bromenn/blank.cfm?ID=70

[76] October 23rd - Oncologist follow-up
http://www.mayoclinic.com/health/cancer/CA00049/
UPDATEAPP=0&SI=2818

[77] October 23rd - Oncologist follow-up Appointment -
Cancer Survival – Recurrence
http://www.mayoclinic.com/health/cancer/CA00049/
UPDATEAPP=0&SI=2818

[79] Letter To My Husband - "In Florence's Own Words"
http://www.inspire.com/groups/lung-cancer-survivors/
discussion/a-litttle-something-to-make-you-smile/

[80] Letter To My Husband - "In Florence's Own Words"
http://www.goodreads.com/author/quotes/3543.Ronald_Reagan
http://quotationsbook.com/quote/46599/#sthash.o1DSsD5O.dpbs

[81] Letter To My Husband - "In Florence's Own Words"
http://www.imdb.com/title/tt0413099/quotes

Glossary Of Terms

While all efforts have been taken to ensure the currency and reliability of the following information, it is important to note that this is not a medical document nor does it constitute medical advice, nor is it a substitute for professional health care.

Anemia: Is defined as a qualitative or quantitative deficiency of hemoglobin, a protein found inside red blood cells (RBCs).

Arimidex: ARIMIDEX (anastrozole) is indicated for the treatment of early or advanced breast cancer in postmenopausal women with hormone receptor-positive disease. ARIMIDEX is the only aromatase inhibitor with conclusive evidence demonstrating superior efficacy and tolerability compared with tamoxifen in both newly diagnosed patients and in those already midway through a course of tamoxifen.

Aromatase Inhibitors: Aromatase inhibitors (AI) are a class of drugs used in the treatment of breast cancer and ovarian cancer in postmenopausal women.
Some cancers require estrogen to grow. Aromatase is an enzyme that synthesizes estrogen. Aromatase inhibitors block the synthesis of estrogen. This lowers the estrogen level, and slows the growth of cancers.

Axillary Lymph Nodes: There are three levels of axillary lymph nodes (the nodes in the underarm or "axilla" area):
1. Level I, the bottom level, below the lower edge of the pectoralis minor muscle.
2. Level II is lying underneath the pectoralis minor muscle.
3. Level III is above the pectoralis minor muscle.
A traditional axillary lymph node dissection usually removes nodes in levels I and II. For women with invasive breast cancer, this procedure accompanies a mastectomy. It may be done at the same time as, or after, a lumpectomy (through a separate incision).

BRCA-1 and BRCA-2: BRCA-1 and BRCA-2 are two genes that are linked with hereditary breast and ovarian cancers. About 200,000 women are diagnosed with invasive breast cancer each year and about 23,000 with ovarian cancer (according to the American Cancer Society). Of these cancers, about 5% to 10% will be due to a mutation in one of the BRCA genes. Men can also inherit an increased risk of developing breast cancer, primarily from an alteration in the BRCA-2 gene.
Individuals with mutations in BRCA1 or BRCA2 have significantly elevated risks for breast cancer (up to 80% lifetime risk), ovarian cancer (up to 40% lifetime risk), bilateral breast cancer and other types of cancers. BRCA mutations are inherited and passed from generation to generation. One half of the time, they are passed from the father's side of the family.

The DNA in white blood cells is used to detect mutations in the BRCA genes. While the gene products (proteins) of the BRCA genes act only in breast and ovarian tissue, the genes are present in every cell of the body and blood is the most easily accessible source of that DNA.

Benign Tumor: A benign tumor is a tumor that lacks all three of the malignant properties of a cancer. Thus, by definition, a benign tumor does not grow in an unlimited, aggressive manner, does not invade surrounding tissues, and does not metastasize.

Biopsy: A biopsy is a medical test involving the removal of cells or tissues for examination. It is the removal of tissue from a living subject to determine the presence or extent of a disease. The tissue is generally examined under a microscope by a pathologist, and can also be analyzed chemically. When an entire lump or suspicious area is removed, the procedure is called an excisional biopsy. When only a sample of tissue is removed with preservation of the histological architecture of the tissue's cells, the procedure is called an incisional biopsy or core biopsy. When a sample of tissue or fluid is removed with a needle in such a way that cells are removed without preserving the histological architecture of the tissue cells, the procedure is called a needle aspiration biopsy.

Bone Scan: A bone scan is a nuclear scanning test to find abnormalities in bone. It is primarily used to diagnose or help diagnose a number of conditions relating to bones, including: cancer of the bone or cancers that have spread (metastasized) to the bone, locating sources of bone pain (e.g. lower back pain) and abnormal bone, diagnosing fractures that may not be seen as easily in traditional X-ray images, and detecting damage to bones due to infection or illness.

Bone Mineral Density (BMD) Test: A bone mineral density test is an easy reliable test that measures the density, or thickness, of your bones. It measures the amount of mineral (calcium) in a specific area of bone. The more mineral you have in the bone measured, the greater your bone density or bone mass (See DEXA Scan).

CA 27.29: Tumor marker. Used in management of breast cancer patients. It is not a screening test for breast cancer.

Carboplatin: Carboplatin is a chemotherapy drug used against some forms of cancer. It was introduced in the late 1980s and has since gained popularity in clinical treatment due to its vastly reduced side-effects compared to its parent compound cisplatin. Cisplatin and carboplatin, as well as oxaliplatin, are classified as DNA alkylating agents.

Central Venous Access Port: The access port device is a plastic tube hooked to a plastic or metal disc called a port. The tube is inserted in either the subclavian or internal jugular vein (major blood vessels under the collarbone) and capped with the port just below the surface of the skin. The port can be used to give medicines and liquids and is also useful for taking blood samples.

Chemotherapy: Chemotherapy, in its most general sense, refers to treatment of disease by chemicals that kill cells, both good and bad, but specifically those of micro-organisms or cancer. In popular usage, it refers to antineoplastic drugs used to treat cancer or the combination of these drugs into a cytotoxic standardized treatment regimen.

CT Scan: Computed tomography (CT) is a medical imaging method employing tomography. Digital geometry processing is used to generate a three-dimensional image of the inside of an object from a large series of two-dimensional X-ray images taken around a single axis of rotation. It is also known as computed axial tomography (CAT or CT scan).

Dexa Scan: Dexa stands for 'Dual Energy X-ray Absorptiometry'. It is the most commonly used test for measuring bone mineral density (See T-Score and Bone Density Test). It is one of the most accurate ways to diagnosis Osteopenia or Osteoporosis (See Osteopenia or Osteoporosis).

Ductal carcinoma in situ (DCIS): Intraductal carcinoma of the breast (Ductal Carcinoma In Situ, DCIS) is the most common type of noninvasive breast cancer in women. Ductal carcinoma refers to the development of cancer cells within the milk ducts of the breast. In situ means "in place" and refers to the fact that the cancer has not moved out of the duct and into any surrounding tissue.

Estrogen Receptor (ER) and Progesterone Receptor (PR): The estrogen receptor (ER) and progesterone receptor (PR) are molecular markers that tell us that the cancer cells can respond to hormonal signals, particularly from estrogen (See Estrogen). The presence of ER and PR on the cancer cells allows us to use hormonal therapies in order to manipulate, or change, the signal to the cancer cells. In simple terms, we can target those receptors ER and PR with hormonal medication. It is quite effective in preventing the spread or recurrence of breast cancer.

Estrogen: Estrogens are a group of steroid compounds, named for their importance in the estrous cycle, and functioning as the primary female sex hormone. Estrogens are used as part of some oral contraceptives, in estrogen replacement therapy of postmenopausal women, and in hormone replacement therapy for trans-women. Like all steroid hormones, estrogens readily diffuse across the cell membrane; inside the cell, they interact with estrogen receptors.

Estrogen Receptor: Estrogen receptor refers to a group of receptors that are activated by the hormone 17ß-estradiol (estrogen). Two types of estrogen receptor exist: ER which is a member of the nuclear hormone family of intracellular receptors and the estrogen G protein coupled receptor GPR30 (GPER), which is a G-protein coupled receptor.

FISH Test: Fluorescence in situ hybridization (FISH) is a test that "maps" the genetic material in a person's cells. This test can be used to visualize specific genes or portions of genes. FISH testing is done on breast cancer tissue removed during biopsy to determine whether the cells have extra copies of the HER2 gene. The more copies of the HER2 gene that are present, the more HER2 receptors the cells have. These HER2 receptors receive signals that stimulate the growth of breast cancer cells.

The FISH test results will tell you that the cancer is either "positive" or "negative" (a result sometimes reported as "zero") for HER2. A positive result suggests that the cancer is likely to respond to treatment with Herceptin (See Herceptin), a treatment that blocks the HER2 receptors from receiving growth signals.

Grading: An important part of evaluating a cancer is to determine its histologic grade. Grade is a marker of how differentiated a cell is. Grade is rated numerically (Grade 1-4) or descriptively (e.g., "high grade" or "low grade"). The higher the numeric grade, the more "poorly differentiated" is the cell, and it is called "high grade". A low-grade cancer has a low number and is "well-differentiated." Grade is most commonly given on a three-tier scale. A cancer that is very poorly differentiated is called anaplastic. Tumors may be graded on four-tier, three-tier, or two-tier scales, depending on the institution and the tumor type.

The tumor grade, along with the staging, is used to develop an individual treatment plan and to predict the patient's prognosis.

Hematocrit: The hematocrit is the proportion of blood volume that is occupied by red blood cells. It is normally about 46% for men and 38% for women. It is considered an integral part of a person's complete blood count results, along with hemoglobin concentration, white blood cell count, and platelet count.

Hemoglobin: Hemoglobin is the red respiratory protein of RBCs that transport oxygen from lungs to tissues. The 2 types of adult hemoglobin are Hb A and Hb A2. Used in diagnosis of anemias.

HER2: HER2, which is also called HER2/neu (See HER2/neu), and HER-2, is the acronym for human epidermal growth factor receptor 2. Knowing your HER2 status is an important part of cancer diagnosis. HER2 is a gene that sends control signals to your cells, telling them to grow, divide, and make repairs. A healthy breast cell has 2 copies of the HER2 gene. Some kinds of breast cancer get started when a breast cell has more than 2 copies of that gene, and those copies start over-producing the HER2 protein. As a result, the affected cells grow and divide much too quickly.

If your breast cancer is tested for HER2 status, the results will be graded as positive or negative. If your results are graded as HER2 positive, that means that your HER2 genes are over-producing the HER2 protein, and that those cells are growing rapidly and creating the cancer. If your results are graded HER2 negative, then the HER2 protein is not causing the cancer.

HER2/neu: HER2/neu stands for "Human Epidermal growth factor Receptor 2" and is a protein giving higher aggressiveness in breast cancers. The protein is found in many human cancers and their excessive signaling may be critical factors in the development and malignancy of tumors. Approximately 15-20 percent of breast cancers have amplification of the HER2/neu gene or over expression of its protein product. Over expression of this receptor in breast cancer is associated with increased disease recurrence and worse prognosis. Because of its prognostic role as well as its ability to predict response to Herceptin breast tumors are routinely checked for over expression of HER2/neu. Over expression of the HER2 gene can be suppressed by the amplification of other genes and the use of the drug Herceptin (See Herceptin).

HER2-positive: HER2-positive breast cancer is a breast cancer that tests positive for a protein called Human Epidermal growth factor Receptor-2 (See HER2), which promotes the growth of cancer cells. About one of every three-breast cancer's the cancer cells make an excess of HER2 due to a gene mutation. This gene mutation can occur in many types of cancer — not only breast cancer.

HER2-positive breast cancers tend to be more aggressive than other types of breast cancer. They're also less responsive to hormone treatment. However, new treatments that specifically target HER2 are proving to be very effective.

Herceptin (Trastuzumab): Herceptin, which specifically targets HER2, kills these cancer cells and decreases the risk of recurrence. Herceptin is often used with chemotherapy. It may also be used alone or in combination with hormone-blocking medications, such as an aromatase inhibitor or tamoxifen. A study published in 2005 found that Herceptin reduce breast cancer recurrence by as much as 50 percent. Herceptin is usually well tolerated, but it does have some potential side effects, such as congestive heart failure and allergic reaction.

Infiltrating ductal carcinoma (IDC): Invasive Ductal Carcinoma (IDC) is a very common type of breast cancer. It starts developing in the milk ducts of your breast, but breaks out of the duct tubes, and invades, or infiltrates, surrounding tissues. Unlike ductal carcinoma in situ (DCIS - see DCIS), which is a non-invasive cancer) IDC is not a well-contained cancer. IDC has the potential to invade your lymph and blood systems, spreading cancer cells to other parts of your body. If IDC spreads beyond its original site, we say it has metastasized (See Metastatic).

Lymph Nodes: A Lymph node is an organ consisting of many types of cells, and is a part of the lymphatic system. Lymph nodes are found all through the body, and act as filters or traps for foreign particles. They contain white blood cells. Thus they are important in the proper functioning of the immune system.

Lymph nodes also have clinical significance. They become inflamed or enlarged in various conditions, which may range from trivial, such as a throat infection, to life threatening such as cancers. In the latter, the condition of lymph nodes is so significant that it is used for cancer staging, which decides the treatment to be employed, and for determining the prognosis.

Lymphedema: Lymphedema, also known as lymphatic obstruction, is a condition of localized fluid retention caused by a compromised lymphatic system.

Lumpectomy: Lumpectomy is a common surgical procedure designed to remove a discrete lump, usually a tumor, benign or otherwise, from an affected man or woman's breast (See WLE). As the tissue removed is generally quite limited and the procedure relatively non-invasive, compared to a mastectomy (See Mastectomy), a lumpectomy is considered a viable means of "breast conservation" or "breast preservation" surgery with all the attendant physical and emotional advantages of such an approach.

Mammary Ductal Carcinoma: Mammary ductal carcinoma is the most common type of breast cancer in women. It comes in two forms: infiltrating ductal carcinoma (IDC), an invasive, malignant and abnormal proliferation of neoplastic cells in the breast tissue and ductal carcinoma in situ (DCIS), a noninvasive, possibly malignant neoplasm that is still confined to the lactiferous ducts, where breast cancer most often originates.

Mammography (Mammogram): The process of using low-dose amplitude-X-rays (usually around 0.7 mSv) to examine the human breast and is used as a diagnostic as well as a screening tool. The goal of mammography is the early detection of breast cancer, typically through detection of characteristic masses and/or micro-calcifications.

Mastectomy: Mastectomy is the medical term for the surgical removal of one or both breasts, partially or completely. Mastectomy is usually done to treat breast cancer (See Lumpectomy/WLE).
Medical oncology and hematology: The American Board of Internal Medicine (ABIM) examines and certifies internists who choose to acquire additional education and training in the dual subspecialty of medical oncology and hematology (the treatment of malignancies of the blood and blood-forming tissues).

Metastatic: Metastatic breast cancer is diagnosed when cells from the original breast tumor have spread beyond your breast to other parts of your body. Even if cancer cells from your breast migrate through your blood stream or lymph system to the lungs, bones, brain, liver, or skin, it is still called breast cancer. Metastatic breast cancer is also called metastatic disease, and is classed as Stage 4 cancer.

Micro-calcifications: Micro-calcifications are tiny specks of mineral deposits (calcium), that can be scattered throughout the mammary gland, or occur in clusters. When found on a mammogram, an operative will then decide whether the specks are of concern - usually, this is not the case. Commonly, they simply indicate the presence of tiny benign cysts, but can signify the presence of early breast cancer; for this reason, it is important to attend regular screening sessions, as recommended by your health provider.

MUGA Scan: A MUGA scan (Multi Gated Acquisition Scan) is a nuclear medicine test to evaluate the function of the heart ventricles. It is also called Radionuclide Angiography. It provides a movie-like image of the beating heart, and allows the doctor to determine the health of the heart's major pumping chambers. The advantages of a MUGA scan is that, it is more accurate than an echocardiogram and it is non-invasive.

Oncologist: Oncologists are physicians who study, diagnose, and treat cancerous tumors. They practice in hospitals and medical centers, university hospitals, and research organizations.

Osteopenia: Osteopenia is a condition where bone mineral density is lower than normal. It is considered by many doctors to be a precursor to osteoporosis. However, not every person diagnosed with osteopenia will develop osteoporosis. More specifically, osteopenia is defined as a bone mineral density T score between -1.0 and -2.5.

Osteoporosis: Osteoporosis is a disease of bone that leads to an increased risk of fracture. In osteoporosis the bone mineral density (BMD) is reduced, bone micro-architecture is disrupted, and the amount and variety of non-collagenous proteins in bone is altered.

Pathologist: Pathologists are physicians who diagnose and characterize disease in living patients by examining biopsies or bodily fluid.

Platelet Count: Platelets are one of the 3 principal components of blood. Platelets play a major role in clotting process. Used in evaluation of bleeding disorders, thrombocytopenia, leukemia and chemotherapeutic management of malignancies.

Progesterone: Progesterone is a C-21 steroid hormone involved in the female menstrual cycle, pregnancy (supports gestation) and embryogenesis of humans and other species. Progesterone belongs to a class of hormones called progestogens, and is the major naturally occurring human progestogen.

Radiation Therapy: Also radiotherapy or radiation oncology is the medical use of ionizing radiation as part of cancer treatment to control malignant cells. This should not to be confused with radiology, the use of radiation in medical imaging and diagnosis.

Radiologist: A physician specialized in radiology, the branch of medicine that uses ionizing and nonionizing radiation for the diagnosis and treatment of disease.

Red Blood Cell Count (RBC): Red blood cells are one of the 3 principal components of blood. The chief function of RBCs is the transporting of oxygen to all parts of the body.

Oncotype DX Test: Oncotype DX is a test that examines a breast cancer patient's tumor tissue at a molecular level, and gives information about her individual disease. This information can help tailor treatment for her breast cancer. Oncotype DX is the first and only gene expression test that has been accepted as demonstrating the ability to predict a patient's benefit from chemotherapy as well as the risk of recurrence.

PET Scan: Positron emission tomography (PET) is a highly specialized imaging technique that uses short-lived radioactive substances to produce three-dimensional colored images of those substances functioning within the body. These images are called PET scans and the technique is termed PET scanning.

Sentinel Lymph Node: The sentinel lymph node is the hypothetical first lymph node or group of nodes reached by metastasizing cancer cells from a tumor. (See Lymph Node)

Sentinel Lymph Node Biopsy: Also known as a sentinel node procedure. This technique is used in the staging of certain types of cancer to see if they have spread to any lymph nodes, since lymph node metastasis is one of the most important prognostic signs.

Staging: The stage of a cancer is a descriptor (usually numbers I to IV) of how much the cancer has spread. The stage often takes into account the size of a tumor, how deep it has penetrated, whether it has invaded adjacent organs, how many lymph nodes it has metastasized to (if any) (See Metastatic), and whether it has spread to distant organs. Staging of cancer is important because the stage at diagnosis is the most powerful predictor of survival, and treatments are often changed based on the stage.

T-Score: The result of your Bone Mineral Density (BMD) test (See Bone Mineral Density Test) is called a T-score. Your T-score compares your bone mass with a population of normal young adult women. The bigger the negative number the lower your bone mass. Example: A T-score of -2.0 means your bone mass is twenty percent below normal. The following chart below helps illustrate what the T-score mean (from a DEXA test only - See DEXA Scan).

Your T-Score: What It Means:
0 to 1.0 Bone mass is normal
-1.0 Bone mass is 10% below normal
-1.5 Bone mass is 15% below normal
-2.0 Bone mass is 20% below normal
You are considered osteoporotic if your bone mass is at least 20% below normal.

Taxotere (Docetaxel): Taxotere is an anti-cancer ("antineoplastic" or "cytotoxic") chemotherapy drug. Taxotere is classified as a "plant alkaloid," a "taxane" and an "antimicrotubule agent."

Tumor: A tumor or tumour is the name for a swelling or lesion formed by an abnormal growth of cells. Tumor is not synonymous with cancer. A tumor can be benign, pre-malignant or malignant, whereas cancer is by definition malignant.

White Blood Cell Count (WBC): White blood cells are one of 3 principal types of blood cells. The principal function of WBCs is to fight infection. Increased levels are often an indication that the body is fighting infection. Decreased levels are common during chemotherapy, and may be an indication of neutropenia.

Wide local excision (WLE): WLE is a surgical procedure to remove a small area of diseased or problematic tissue with a margin of normal tissue (See Lumpectomy). This procedure is commonly performed on the breast and to skin lesions, but can be used on any area of the body (See Lumpectomy). The tissue removed is examined under a microscope to confirm the type of lesion and to grade malignant tumors. This examination also determines if the lesion has been removed without leaving any behind. The results of a WLE will determine any future treatments if needed.

Venous Access Port: This device is a plastic tube hooked to a plastic or metal disc called a port. The tube is inserted in either the subclavian or internal jugular vein (major blood vessels under the collarbone) and capped with the port just below the surface of the skin. The port can be used to give medicines and liquids and is also useful for taking blood samples.

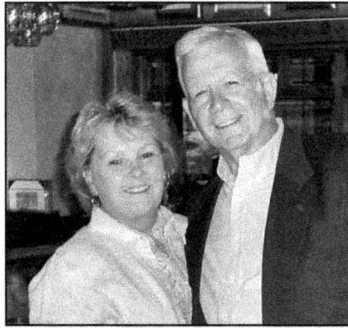

G.P. Carbonneau and his wife,
Florence a six year cancer
survivor.

Mr. Carbonneau is the recipient of the State of Florida Rehabilitation Association's Achievement Award. He has developed computer-based applications for the National Cryptology School applying expertise in Computer Sciences and Instructional Design.

Mr. Carbonneau has served as a proposal reviewer consultant for the National Science Foundation, Small Business Innovative Research program. He holds two United States patents in computer related peripheral communication terminals. He has been featured in Who's Who in Technology Today, Computer Sciences and Forbes Magazine, "Faces Behind the Figures." Authored and published a fictional novel titled ADX prompted by personal experience with federal and local agencies.

www.ingramcontent.com/pod-product-compliance
Lightning Source LLC
Chambersburg PA
CBHW072124270326
41931CB00010B/1664